NURSE EDUCATOR COMPETENCIES:
CREATING AN EVIDENCE-BASED
PRACTICE FOR NURSE EDUCATORS

Judith A. Halstead
DNS, RN, ANEF
Editor

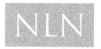

National League
for **Nursing**

National League for Nursing
61 Broadway
New York, NY 10006
212-363-5555 or 800-669-1656
www.nln.org

ISBN 9781934758380

Cover design by Brian Vigorita
Director or Marketing Communications, Laerdal Medical Corporation

Printed in the United States of America   9 8 7

NURSE EDUCATOR COMPETENCIES:
CREATING AN EVIDENCE-BASED PRACTICE FOR NURSE EDUCATORS

CREATING AN EVIDENCE-BASED PRACTICE FOR NURSE EDUCATORS

TABLE OF CONTENTS

The health care system depends on well-prepared nurses and graduates from schools of nursing to provide safe and effective nursing care. Advances in understanding how students learn, ubiquitous educational technology, proliferation of new types of academic programs, and national recommendations for interdisciplinary learning all point to the need for change in our current teaching practices. Nurse educators must, therefore, understand not only the needs of the health care system and clinical nursing care, but also must acquire the knowledge, skills and abilities that are requisite for teaching nursing in complex educational environments.

Nurse educators must be prepared to understand the needs of the learner; facilitate learning; socialize students to the profession; evaluate learning outcomes; assure employers that graduates can provide safe patient care; design educational programs; provide leadership for change; develop their own careers within the educational environment; and contribute to the scholarship and research that advance the science of nursing education. *Nurse Educator Competencies: Creating an Evidence-based Practice for Nurse Educators* offers nurses a framework for developing these competencies which are required for assuming the role and responsibilities of nurse educator.

The educator competencies framework offered in this book serves several purposes. First, the framework can be used to guide the development of curricula in master's, post-master's, doctoral, and continuing education programs that are designed to prepare future nurse educators. These competencies also constitute a plan for role development for current educators or a guide for self-directed and continued learning for current or aspiring educators who seek to improve their teaching practice and develop their careers as nurse educators. The competencies also can be viewed as an assessment framework, serving as a foundation for individual career development plans or certifying to the public that a nurse educator has attained the requisite skills, knowledge and abilities for advanced practice as a nurse educator.

This book, the result of several years of scholarly work by master nurse educators, is at once a guide, a blueprint, and a mandate for developing fully the advanced practice role of nurse educator. Students, colleagues, and patients deserve competent nurse educators. This book provides a framework for developing this competence.

Diane M. Billings, EdD, RN, FAAN
Chancellor's Professor Emeritus
Indiana University School of Nursing
Indianapolis, Indiana
July 2007

CREATING AN EVIDENCE-BASED PRACTICE FOR NURSE EDUCATORS

This book is an outcome of the work of the National League for Nursing's Task Group on Nurse Educator Competencies. It provides the reader with a comprehensive synthesis of research literature related to educator competencies which led to the development of the NLN Core Competencies for Nurse Educators. In the relatively short time that has elapsed since the publication of the Core Competencies in 2005, the nursing profession has already experienced the positive impact of these competencies on nurse educator preparation and development.

Throughout the United States, the educator competencies are being used to guide the development of graduate nursing programs designed to prepare future nursing faculty. They served as the test blueprint for the development of the NLN certification examination for nurse educators. The core competencies are being used to help define the roles and responsibilities of nurse educators in various educational settings, thereby assisting with recruitment and retention efforts in nursing education. And finally, doctoral students are using the core competencies in their research studies to further explicate the knowledge, skills and attitudes nurse educators need to effectively teach learners to practice in today's complex health care settings.

Chapter One describes the process used by the task group to conduct the literature review and develop the competencies with their accompanying task statements. This chapter also addresses the significance of the core competencies to nursing education and the nursing profession. Chapters Two through Nine are devoted to each of the eight core competencies, with each chapter organized to present the synthesis of the research literature for that specific competency, research gaps that were evident in the literature during the years (1992 – 2004) covered by this review, and questions that can be used to guide future research efforts on the role of nurse educators. Chapter Ten provides concluding comments on the impact the core competencies will have on advancing the science of nursing education.

The literature that is synthesized in this book clearly illustrates the complexity of our roles as nurse educators, the challenges that face us, and the rewards that are associated with teaching the future stewards of our profession. Nurse educators, novice and expert alike, as well as students engaged in graduate study will find the book to be a helpful resource to their own scholarship related to the educator role.

Judith A. Halstead, DNS, RN, ANEF
July, 2007

CREATING AN EVIDENCE-BASED PRACTICE FOR NURSE EDUCATORS

ACKNOWLEDGMENTS

I would like to acknowledge the many individuals who worked collaboratively to conduct, analyze, and synthesize the literature review that is presented in this book and informed the development of the *NLN Core Competencies for Nurse Educators and Task Statements*. The members of the Task Group for Nurse Educator Competencies are dedicated nurse educators and scholars who worked voluntarily for more than two years on this project, contributing an untold number of hours. You will find each of their names listed on the contributor page. I thank them for the spirit of inquiry, scholarship, enthusiasm, creativity, and team work that they unfailingly brought to the work the task group was charged to complete.

I would also like to thank Martha Scheckel, PhD, RN, who provided assistance to the Task Group in structuring and organizing the early stages of the literature review. And finally, I also want to acknowledge and gratefully thank the NLN staff who supported the work of the Task Group and were a consistent source of inspiration to its members -- Dr. Mary Anne Rizzolo and Dr. Terry Valiga.

CREATING AN EVIDENCE-BASED PRACTICE FOR NURSE EDUCATORS

CHAPTER ONE
DEVELOPMENT OF THE CORE COMPETENCIES OF NURSE EDUCATORS

This book reflects the work of the National League for Nursing's Task Group on Nurse Educator Competencies, which was begun in 2002 and completed in 2004. The comprehensive review and synthesis of the literature that the task group completed resulted in the development of the nurse educator competencies that are described in this publication.

The development of nurse educator competencies is a significant contribution to nursing education and the nursing profession. It has been well documented that the nursing profession is facing a serious shortage of nurse educators. The aging population of nursing faculty, increased use of part-time faculty, and the relatively high number of nurse educators who are not doctorally prepared are faculty trends that have been reported by the National League for Nursing (2002a). Because of the decreased number of graduate programs that are specifically designed to prepare nurse educators, there are also relatively few nurses in the pipeline who are prepared to assume the educator role and replace the large number of nursing faculty scheduled to retire in the next ten to fifteen years.

The consequences of this impending shortage of nurse educators are serious for our profession. Schools of nursing are reporting that qualified applicants are being denied admission due to a lack of qualified faculty. In addition to this immediate concern, the profession must also be concerned about the loss of nursing education expertise that will occur as faculty in all types of nursing programs retire over the next decade. The profession must now focus attention on developing the next generation of nurse educators. It is essential that those who teach are well prepared to do so, and that they engage in an evidence-based practice of teaching. There is an increased interest in higher education on the scholarship of teaching, and the importance of preparing faculty to assume the role of "teacher" is being acknowledged by the academy. We need to ensure that the educators of the future are effective and have the competencies needed to facilitate learning in an increasingly complex health care environment. The nurse educator competencies described in this book provide a framework that identifies the knowledge, skills, and attitudes required to successfully implement the educator role in a variety of settings.

The genesis of the nurse educator competencies can be found in the discussions that occurred among expert educators who formed the Think Tank on Graduate Education Preparation for the Nurse Educator Role that was convened by the National League for Nursing in December 2001. The think tank, chaired by Dr. M. Louise Fitzpatrick, was composed of individuals who were expert educators in nursing and higher education, knowledgeable in graduate education, and represented a variety of institutions and backgrounds, including academia and staff development. One outcome of the work of the think tank was the NLN Position Statement on The Preparation of Nurse Educators (2002b).

In the course of discussions, the think tank members addressed the question, "What do educators need to know, or be able to do, to implement the role successfully and effectively?" This question was discussed within the framework of different environments – comprehensive universities, liberal arts colleges, community colleges, research-intensive environments, and clinical settings. The continuum of educator roles – from the novice educator who primarily focuses on the teaching role to the expert educator who assumes responsibility for designing and implementing program curricula – was also discussed. From these discussions, a draft of competencies for nurse educators was developed.

When the Task Group on Nurse Educator Competencies was charged with its mission, the group was asked to build upon the initial work of the Think Tank on Graduate Education Preparation for the Nurse Educator Role, to validate and further develop the proposed competencies that had emerged from the think tank discussions. The specific activities of the task group were to: 1) conduct a comprehensive review of the literature related to educator competencies; 2) formulate competencies for nurse educators based upon the literature review; 3) identify gaps in the body of knowledge about educator competencies; and 4) identify priorities for future research efforts related to educator competencies.

The task group conducted a review of literature published between the years of 1992 and 2004, focusing primarily on research literature in nursing, higher education, medicine, allied health, social work, psychology, and sociology databases. It was the goal of the task group to produce an evidence-based report on educator competencies; however, in some competency areas there was little research reported in the literature. In those instances, the task group had to draw more heavily from non-research-based literature, drawing upon best practices and exemplars. The resulting competency statements were developed by the task group and have been subsequently revised to their current form based upon further review and feedback from nurse educators across the country.

The future impact of the nurse educator competencies on the nursing profession is significant. Nurse educators who understand the educational process, and embrace it as a scholarly endeavor, will be the profession's leaders in building a science of nursing education. Furthermore, educators who are well prepared for the role will influence undergraduate and graduate curriculum and program development to produce strong graduates prepared to engage in clinical practice, pursue advanced education, and engage in scholarship that builds upon the existing body of nursing knowledge.

Specifically, these competencies provide direction for the development of graduate programs that prepare nurse educators. The competencies provide a framework for curriculum development and program design by identifying the essential knowledge, skills, and attitudes relevant to the educator role. The competencies can also be used to guide workplace recruitment and retention activities as they comprehensively define the roles and responsibilities of the educator for those who may wish to assume the role. This is essential to recruiting qualified individuals to educator positions. It is important to note, however, that there is **not** the expectation that all educators possess all the competencies in their totality. The educator's level of experience and the institutional setting will greatly impact the expected competencies in the role. For example, what is expected of the novice educator in a community college is vastly different than what is expected of the senior educator in a research-intensive university. The competencies can be used to focus faculty development efforts that will help facilitate growth along the continuum that exists within the educator role.

The nurse educator competencies also provide direction for public policy efforts. They can be used to support funding initiatives for the preparation of nurse educators and can also help identify the "right" mix of faculty for a given institutional environment. Finally, the competencies can be used to guide scholarship efforts related to the educator role. This book identifies research priorities for the future that can further define the role of the nurse educator.

The challenges that face nursing education are many. To maintain a strong cadre of practicing professionals, it is critical that the nursing profession address the shortage of qualified educators. The competencies of nurse educators clearly illustrate the richness and complexity of the educator role. As the nursing profession confronts the challenge of who will be the nurse educators of the future, these competencies for nurse educators can be used as a framework by which we design a preferred future for nursing education.

References

National League for Nursing (2002a). *Nurse educators 2002 – Report of the faculty census survey of RN and graduate programs.* New York: Author.

National League for Nursing (2002b). *NLN position statement on the preparation of nurse educators.* New York: Author.

CREATING AN EVIDENCE-BASED PRACTICE FOR NURSE EDUCATORS

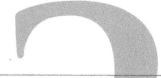

CHAPTER TWO
FACILITATE LEARNING

Learning in nursing education takes place within a broad spectrum of academic and practice domains. The nurse educator's role in facilitating learning is complex, multifaceted, and includes an appreciation of the interwoven nature of teaching and learning. To be effective, nurse educators must develop a personal teaching style, use a variety of teaching methods, and demonstrate content knowledge and professional practice expertise. In other words, nurse educators must understand the content they are teaching as well as the pedagogical issues related to teaching a practice discipline. This includes having an understanding of the contemporary issues in the discipline and the best ways of effectively engaging students in learning about them. To paraphrase the words of Ernest Boyer (1990), nurse educators must be able to transform and extend knowledge, as well as transmit it.

The following competency statements include the knowledge, skills, and attitudes nurse educators must develop in order to facilitate learning effectively. The nurse educator:

- Implements a variety of teaching strategies appropriate to learner needs, desired learner outcomes, content, and context

- Grounds teaching strategies in educational theory and evidence-based teaching practices

- Recognizes multicultural, gender, and experiential influences on teaching and learning

- Engages in self-reflection and continued learning to improve teaching practices that facilitate learning

- Uses information technologies skillfully to support the teaching-learning process

- Practices skilled oral, written, and electronic communication that reflects an awareness of self and others, along with an ability to convey ideas in a variety of contexts

- Models critical and reflective thinking

- Creates opportunities for learners to develop their critical thinking and clinical reasoning skills

- Shows enthusiasm for teaching, learning, and nursing that inspires and motivates students

- Demonstrates interest in and respect for learners

- Uses personal attributes (e.g., caring, confidence, patience, integrity, and flexibility) that facilitate learning

- Develops collegial working relationships with students, faculty, colleagues, and clinical agency personnel to promote positive learning environments

- Maintains the professional practice knowledge base needed to help learners prepare for contemporary nursing practice

- Serves as a role model of professional nursing

Review of the Literature

This review summarizes and synthesizes the literature related to the educator's role in facilitating learning, with an emphasis on research literature. The main focus of the literature review was the educator qualities that characterize effective teaching and that facilitate learning. Clinical teaching and the role of the preceptor, which present unique challenges with regard to facilitating learning, are also reviewed. Most of the studies reviewed were surveys yielding descriptive data. In addition, the vast majority reflected the behavioral model of education. The studies' methodologies included quantitative methods (i.e., questionnaires), qualitative methods (i.e., individual and focus group interviews), or a mix of the two methodologies.

Effective Teaching

Effective teaching was addressed in the literature from the perspectives of students, teachers, and administrators. Within the literature reviewed, the characteristics of general teaching effectiveness that were addressed were: developing a personal teaching style, knowing and using a variety of teaching methods, and demonstrating knowledge of the content taught.

Developing a Personal Teaching Style. Many authors described the importance of the educator's interpersonal skills in facilitating learning. Lowman (1995) described the skills necessary for masterful teaching as having two dimensions: 1) creating intellectual excitement, which includes knowing and presenting content and stimulating the emotions associated with intellectual activity, and 2) developing interpersonal rapport, both psychological and emotional, that reflects respect for the student. Campbell (1997), while researching award-winning teachers' personal constructions of the teaching process, concluded that there may be "a psychological developmental aspect to the development of effective teachers" since teachers' construction of teaching goals, relationships with students, content, and context all shift in parallel with "established schema for epistemological and intellectual development" (p. 394). Trow (1994) also described teaching as relational, as a process consisting of "emotional and intellectual connection between teacher and learner." (p. 72). Harris (1998) labeled one category of teacher effectiveness as "artistry," to acknowledge that teaching is a personal, creative, reflective enterprise of sustained professional development.

Some researchers have made distinctions between personality traits and interpersonal style. For instance, Whitehead (1997) described five major categories that characterize effective clinical and theory nursing instructors: interpersonal relationships, personality traits, teaching practices, knowledge and experience, and evaluation procedures. For purposes of this review the first two categories, personality traits and interpersonal style, are considered together and referred to generally as personal style.

Characteristics of effective college and university teachers that reflect personal style included motivating students to do their best, creating a comfortable learning atmosphere, communicating effectively, and showing concern for student learning (Young & Shaw,

1999). Wills' (1997) survey of nursing students regarding what helps them learn indicated interpersonal relationship skills and personal traits of the teacher were two factors of great importance to students. Similarly, in a study conducted in the United Kingdom, Camiah (1998) rated effective communication and interpersonal skills as important educational management skills for new clinical nurse tutors (teachers). The ability to motivate students, as well as being caring and inspirational, friendly and approachable, being committed and showing excitement and enthusiasm for teaching were all characteristics of exemplary professors as rated by master's level business and education students (Hill, 1995).

Waring (1996) surveyed students, effective teachers, and supervisors of teachers in an adult education program and reported that characteristics of these effective teachers included showing enthusiasm for teaching and the subject, respect and concern for the students, and patience. In addition, these teachers reflected self-assurance in their teaching, and modeled their teaching style after their own effective teachers. Kelly (2002) also noted the importance of teacher self-efficacy in providing motivation for teaching and teaching effectiveness.

The personal style of the teacher is important in online, asynchronous education as well. Specifically addressing online education, Milstead and Nelson (1998) noted that personal characteristics contributing to effective teaching with online nursing courses include flexibility and patience, and "an ability to project a warm online persona" (p. 7). The American Association of Colleges of Nursing's (AACN, 2000) White Paper on Distance Education noted that faculty who are engaged in distance education need to possess creativity, flexibility, and a willingness to learn new teaching strategies. In face-to-face interactions with students, teachers can model the personal traits of compassion, caring, patience, and sensitivity to help students learn how to relate well to others. These traits may be more difficult to model online. Interestingly, Nesler, Hanner, Melburg and McGowan (2001) reported that baccalaureate nursing students graduating from distance education programs had significantly ($p < .01$) better professional socialization outcomes than students graduating from traditional campus-based programs. The researchers used two different socialization measures in this study; only one of the measures, the Nursing Care Role Orientation Scale, had satisfactory psychometric properties.

Reflecting on one's own teaching also influences teaching effectiveness. Reflection is presented as a personal teaching style in some research findings and as a specific teaching methodology in others. Harris (1998) described reflection as a component of teaching artistry (personal style), whereas Clarke and James (1993) described and encouraged the use of different types of reflecting in a self-study program for teachers specifically striving to be effective teachers by developing an understanding of the learning process. Similarly, in a case study, Johnston and Tinning (2001) described a group reflective practice strategy for developing facilitators of problem-based learning (PBL) in nursing curricula. This strategy consisted of establishing a discussion group of PBL facilitators that focused on discussing generic PBL scenarios and also promoted sharing of personal performance issues with PBL.

Another example of using reflection to improve one's teaching was provided by Pinsky and Irby (1997) in their survey of physicians who teach clinical medicine. Pinsky and Irby asked forty master clinical teachers to provide examples of how a teaching failure had made them a better teacher. The authors described the three phases of teaching as being planning, teaching, and reflection. Reflection-on-action, which occurs after teaching has taken place, can help teachers evaluate and plan future teaching activities. The respondents in this study indicated that reflection-on-action revealed that teaching failures had typically occurred because of flawed implementation plans or the selection of a wrong teaching strategy. By using reflection to evaluate their teaching, these master teachers were able to capitalize upon teaching failures to help ensure future teaching successes. Self-reflection on their teaching was also a characteristic of outstanding adult education teachers who had subject-matter knowledge but who lacked teacher preparation (Waring, 1996).

Knowing and Using a Variety of Teaching Methods. Knowing and using a variety of teaching methods that engage the learner is another aspect of being an effective teacher. In a classic article, Chickering and Gamson (1987) identified seven principles for good teaching practice in undergraduate education as: encouraging contact between students and faculty, developing reciprocity and cooperation among students, encouraging active learning, giving prompt feedback, emphasizing time on task, communicating high expectations, and respecting diverse talents and ways of learning. These principles emphasize how teachers practice teaching rather than focus on what they teach (content). Designing and implementing teaching strategies that emphasize these seven principles helps the teacher meet learners' needs.

Camiah (1998) advocated for new clinical nursing tutors in the United Kingdom to use a variety of teaching methods that would facilitate the progression of students in their knowledge and skill acquisition as practitioners. Kelly (2002) noted that using teaching strategies that build on students' past experiences, stimulate thinking, emphasize problem solving, and motivate students to learn fosters higher levels of thinking. In essence, knowledge of teaching and learning theories provides an excellent framework for facilitating learning. Based upon a review of the educational literature, Harris (1998) concluded that the best teaching method is a mixture of teaching methodologies that are suited to the learning context.

Having a philosophy of teaching and learning that reflects a student-centered approach and a willingness to learn new skills and teaching strategies is important to effective teaching and applies to e-learning and distance education, as well as traditional classroom teaching (AACN, 2000; Cobb & Billings, 2000; Milstead & Nelson, 1998; Sherman, 1998). Sherman noted that teachers must be able to facilitate the sampling and interpretation of materials and to act as coaches in guiding students as they transform information gleaned directly from electronic databases. In a study of nursing teachers and students who interacted online,

Nosek (2003) reported that in order for teachers to be successful at facilitating learning in online courses they need to be open to learning from students and changing how they teach.

In a review of the research literature in higher education, Adams (2002) reported that colleges and universities want new faculty who can develop courses that integrate technology and incorporate civic engagement; multicultural, international, and interdisciplinary learning experiences; and writing. New teachers are expected to be knowledgeable about technology, active learning, field-based learning, and diversity; use creative strategies that engage students; and embrace pedagogies that include collaborative learning, simulations, and field experiences. DeNeef (2002) reported in an evaluation of the Preparing Future Faculty Program (PFFP) that alumni of this program were more likely to be familiar with a range of teaching strategies, classroom issues, and teaching resources, which served them well in their first teaching positions. Alumni of the PFFP also reported feeling prepared to handle many different teaching situations.

Several authors have described effective teaching behaviors for educators. Diekelmann (2001) described narrative pedagogy, a research-based pedagogy arising from nursing education for nurse teachers, students, and clinicians that utilizes conventional, phenomenological, critical, and feminist pedagogies along with postmodern discourse, as one teaching methodology that is effective in facilitating learning. Whitehead (1997), in her study on the characteristics of effective clinical and classroom educators in an associate degree nursing program, stated that nurse educators should have a good understanding of theories of adult learning and be taught effective teaching behaviors. Similarly, Hewlett (1993) described the importance of nurse educators knowing adult learning principles and strategies to become competent facilitators of adult learning. In a study conducted in the Netherlands to identify the profiles of medical school tutors (teachers) ($N = 67$) who effectively use problem-based learning, DeGrave, Dolmans, and van der Vleuten (1999) divided tutors into two groups, with one group focused more on facilitating the learning process and the other group focused more on using expert knowledge. Tutors stressing process were rated by students as more effective than those stressing content. Tutors rated as most effective scored high on each of four dimensions of behavior as measured by the Tutor Intervention Profile (TIP): elaborating upon and stimulating discussion, directing the learning process, integrating knowledge, and stimulating interaction and individual accountability. Construct validity of the TIP instrument was established; reliability of the instrument was not addressed.

In separate research studies involving business students, both Kaiser (2000) and Tang (1997) addressed teaching attributes that contribute to teaching effectiveness. The highest effectiveness ratings were for teachers who presented material clearly, provided helpful feedback, chose relevant content, were knowledgeable, showed concern for learning, and used appropriate evaluation methods (Kaiser, 2000). In a study of 6,395 undergraduate and graduate student evaluations of 126 business faculty at a state university in the southeastern United States, Tang used multiple regression to identify the most important factors that predict teaching effectiveness of faculty: presents material clearly, answers students' questions, appears well prepared for class, and treats students courteously and professionally.

Utilizing Chickering and Gamson's (1987) seven principles of effective teaching, as well as two additional principles related to subject-matter expertise and organization as a framework for their study, Thompson and Scheckley (1997) described the differences in classroom teaching preferences of adult BSN students (N = 64 RNs), adult non-nurse students (N = 36), and traditional BSN students (N = 106) from four different nursing programs. The researchers developed an instrument to measure effective teaching practices that was adapted from two previously existing surveys. The reliability and validity of the adapted instrument were established for this study with the instrument being determined to have content validity and acceptable internal reliability. Factor analyses of the students' responses indicated that four factors related to teacher attributes were stable across time when describing a "best" classroom learning experience: being organized and knowledgeable; clarifying time on task; encouraging cooperative learning, and promoting active learning. In addition to these four factors, they also found that a teacher who communicated high expectations contributed to a positive classroom learning experience. Students evaluated a classroom learning experience as poor if the four "best" classroom factors were not present, if student-teacher interactions were not facilitated, and if diverse ways of learning were not addressed. Students from all categories tended to agree about factors contributing to "poor" classroom experiences. Interestingly, prior work experience with the subject matter had more of an impact on student learning preferences than did age, with returning RNs valuing cooperative and active learning more than adult non-RNs or traditional college-age students. These results led the researchers to conclude that adult learners may have different learning needs that are not accounted for by age alone. They recommended replication of the study with a larger sample size.

There were numerous studies of specific approaches to teaching or effective teaching strategies reported in the literature. In one study, six categories of competencies for teaching small groups of medical students were identified and validated – teaching orientation, motivating, presenting, clarifying, elaborating and consolidating, and confirming (Preston-Whyte, Clark, Petersen, & Fraser, 1999). Beeson and Kring (1999) reported that students who were taught blood pressure measurement using traditional lecture and linear video had significantly more factual knowledge than did students who were taught by interactive video; however, there were no significant differences in the performance of blood pressure measurement between the two groups. In a mixed method study in the United Kingdom, Mhaolrunaigh and Clifford (1998) addressed the use of shared learning environments in which nurses preparing to be teachers learn from each other. While the student teachers felt they learned in a shared learning environment, they did not feel prepared to transfer the use of this teaching methodology to their own practice as nurse educators. The authors identified the importance of preparing educators to become effective facilitators of shared learning; however, no definitive recommendations for teacher preparation were offered by the researchers. Knight (2001), in addressing effective teaching strategies for social work instructors, indicated educators can help students learn by demonstrating knowledge about student field experiences, helping students apply theory in practice situations, organizing learning experiences, and serving as professional role models.

Several authors addressed educator competencies related to the use of technology in education. Nurse educators who self-reported competence in computer literacy skills were more likely to incorporate use of computers in the classroom (Austin, 1999). Thach and Murphy (1995) identified roles and specific competencies needed for distance education professionals who work with faculty and staff to develop distance education programs. These competencies included strong communication skills, the ability to collaborate, and the ability to provide constructive feedback to others. Saranto and Tallberg (1998) reported that many nurse educators are not familiar with nursing education software and lack confidence in their own abilities in computer-assisted education. These same authors also reported that the information systems used in practice settings are not readily available to nurse educators, thus affecting the educators' competence with using these systems. If nurse educators do not feel competent using technology or information systems, this has potentially serious implications for adequately preparing students to practice in information-based health care systems.

Non-research articles also addressed educator competence with using a variety of teaching strategies. Link and Scholtz (2000) advocated that faculty must be proficient in using technology tools: email, word processing, and software applications for online course development and management. Billings (1995) described one nursing school's plan for faculty development in computer technologies and identified computer competencies for nursing faculty that included basic competencies (such as formatting disks and using a computer); tool skill competencies (such as word processing, spreadsheets, literature search, and statistical software); communication competencies (such as electronic mail, World Wide Web, and computer conferencing), and teaching competencies (such as desktop publishing, using computer-based instruction, computer-administered testing, and presentation graphics). Marashio (1995) described how to design questions to promote student thinking, suggesting that teachers critically evaluate all the educational tools they use to discover whether they are indeed helping or h indering student learning. Zimmermann (2003) summarized tips for effective teaching, including being focused on the learner, using of a variety of teaching methods, utilizing silence to allow the learner to reflect, and repeating relevant content.

Demonstrating Knowledge of the Content Taught. While many studies identified knowledge of subject matter as an essential prerequisite for effective teaching, a few studies specifically addressed faculty competence with content areas thought to be essential for inclusion in nursing curricula. For example, Shoultz and Amundson (1998) surveyed nurse educators' (N = 191) from six different educational institutions about their knowledge of and skills in primary health care. They reported that the subjects had more knowledge about primary health care than the researchers had anticipated, and that educators who had more knowledge used significantly more active teaching strategies than educators with less knowledge about primary health care.

Murphy, Scott, and Mandel (1996) conducted a longitudinal study of nursing faculty fellows (N = 35) in ten schools of nursing who had participated in a faculty development program funded by the National Institute on Alcohol Abuse and Alchoholism and the National Institute on Drug Abuse to determine what substance abuse content areas these faculty felt were important to include in undergraduate and graduate nursing curricula. Content validity and reliability was established for the researcher-developed questionnaire used to measure faculty responses. The findings of this longitudinal study indicated that the faculty fellows' knowledge of substance abuse remained stable over time and resulted in the identification of substance abuse content appropriate for undergraduate and graduate curricula.

In a survey of 266 baccalaureate and higher degree nursing programs, McNeil et al. (2003) described information technology skills being taught by nursing faculty, including information literacy skills and use of the Internet (50% or more of programs surveyed), use of email (35% of programs), database applications (31% of programs) and spreadsheet applications (27% of programs). Despite the fact that many programs included information technology content, survey results indicated that faculty were not necessarily prepared to teach this content. Thirty-nine percent (39%) of the programs rated faculty at the advanced beginner level of preparation for using and teaching information technology content and skills; 18% rated faculty as novices; 29% of programs rated faculty at the competent level; and only 13% of the programs rated their faculty as being expert with information technology.

The findings of these studies appear to support the assertion that when faculty possess specific knowledge and skills related to the content they are teaching, the learning environment will be positively affected and result in the use of more active teaching strategies. At a time when many nurse educators report being given teaching assignments in content areas outside their areas of expertise, it is important to understand how this practice can compromise the quality of the students' educational experience.

Other non-evidence-based articles supported the need for teachers to be knowledgeable about specific teaching approaches within an area of specialized knowledge. For example, Thomas (1992) advocated for a feminist pedagogical approach to teaching women's health and Jackson and Sullivan (1999) described a teaching innovation using the arts and humanities to help midwifery students explore a range of human concerns related to parenting and family concerns. In addition, Thompson (2002) identified competencies for midwifery teachers when teaching students, including knowledge of adult learning theory, use of multiple teaching strategies, and how to develop learning plans, basing these competencies upon a philosophy of midwifery values and model of care.

Clinical Teaching

The research studies of the clinical nurse educator role that were reviewed for this book focused primarily on effective clinical teaching in undergraduate education. Effective clinical teaching in graduate nursing education has not received as much attention in the research literature. The identified areas of educator expertise in clinical teaching were consistent throughout the literature: clinical competence; teaching competence; interpersonal skills or relationships with students, and the educators' intrapersonal characteristics.

Studies related to characteristics of the effective clinical nurse educator have reported variable findings. In a study conducted among undergraduate students (N = 123) enrolled in three Israeli schools of nursing, Benor and Leviyof (1997) determined that clinical nursing competence, student evaluation methods, teaching skills, and interpersonal characteristics were ranked in descending order as the most important characteristics of a competent clinical teacher. Least important appeared to be characteristics related to the teacher's personality. There were some significant differences in the rankings, though, based upon the experience level of the students, with less experienced students ranking student evaluation methods higher than clinical competence, and more experienced students reversing the rank order of those two characteristics.

In contrast to Benor and Leviyof's (1997) findings, Wills (1997), citing Wong (1978), indicated that less experienced students valued how they were treated by faculty as most important, which suggests that interpersonal skills may be more important when teaching more junior nursing students. In a study conducted in an Australian university school of nursing, Lee, Cholowski, and Williams (2002) also reported that less experienced students ranked items related to interpersonal relationships higher than did more experienced students.

Nahas, Nour, and Al-Nobani (1999) examined Jordanian nursing students' perceptions of effective clinical educators. In this descriptive study of the perceptions of undergraduate nursing students (N = 452), results indicated that the professional competence of the educator was the most important characteristic of an effective clinical educator. The researchers acknowledged that this finding was different from similar studies that had been conducted in Western countries (i.e., Australia, the United States, and the United Kingdom) and raised the question of cultural differences. Given the increasing diversity in society, it would appear that the influence of the sociocultural context in which clinical education occurs is an important area for nursing education researchers to pursue.

In the years covered by this review (1992-2004), there was no evidence of research in the literature that addressed the clinical teaching competencies required at the graduate level of nursing education. However, in graduate nursing education, clinical preceptors are commonly used to facilitate student learning in the practice setting and the role of the preceptor has received some attention in the literature. The role of the preceptor is addressed in the final section of this review.

Several studies were found that focus on role expectations of clinical nurse educators, including the rights and the responsibilities of the position. Specific categories of clinical educator skills or competencies have been described by Whitman (1990) and by Bergman and Gaitskill (1990). The purpose of Whitman's exploratory study, which used the Delphi technique, was to identify teaching behaviors of the clinical teacher that might be evaluated by clinical peers. Whitman organized the competencies for clinical nurse educators into three skills categories – nursing, interpersonal, and instructional. With the use of a three-round Delphi, consensus was reached by faculty and clinical peers on specific behaviors for each category that were identified as very important for clinical educators. Bergman and Gaitskill identified three slightly different domains of competence required for clinical teaching: professional competence; relationships with students, and personal attributes. The discussion in the next section of this review is organized according to those same three domains of clinical teaching competencies.

Demonstrating Professional Clinical Competence. Bergman and Gaitskill (1990) described professional clinical competencies of nurse educators as: showing genuine interest in patients and their care, being well informed and able to communicate knowledge to students, and demonstrating skills, attitudes, and values that are to be developed by the student in the clinical area. Nurse educators need to maintain clinical competence to teach in the clinical setting and to serve as role models for students.

Two studies related to clinical competence of nurse educators were conducted in the United Kingdom. Both of these studies raised questions about the educator's role in the practice setting. Goorapah (1997) investigated nurse teachers' and clinicians' perceptions of what constituted clinical credibility and clinical competence. He interviewed a total of 20 teachers (N = 10) and clinicians (N = 10). Findings indicated that while clinical credibility was more vaguely defined by the participants than clinical competence, the two concepts were perceived to be similar. However, the clinicians did tend to define competence and credibility as being related to the actual delivery of "hands-on" care, while teachers were much broader in their interpretation of the terms. Goorapah raised the question as to what extent it is realistic to expect nurse teachers to be clinically competent and credible when they do not practice extensively in clinical settings and called for establishing clarity of the nurse teachers' role. Davies, White, Riley, and Twinn (1996) focused their study on the role of the nurse teacher in practice settings. Interviewing teachers, practitioners, and students, the researchers primarily sought to clarify the role of the teacher on the practice team in order to more effectively help students learn in the clinical setting. It emerged from the interviews that nurse teachers may need to determine where their time would be better spent – teaching students themselves or teaching practitioners how to best teach students.

The studies of Sieh and Bell (1994), Brown, Forrest and Pollock (1998) and Gignac-Caille and Oermann (2001) indicated that teacher credibility depends on clinical competence, the demonstration of specialist knowledge in a particular setting, judgment, and preparation for the clinical experience. Whitman (1990) identified technical, assessment, and communication skills, and meeting a patient's physical and psychosocial needs as important nursing skills for the educator, as well as displaying behaviors that demonstrate knowledge. Sieh and Bell also stated that the clinical nurse educator must take responsibility for his or her own actions, and be well prepared for teaching.

In addition to the previously described studies conducted in the United Kingdom, the professional nursing competence of clinical nurse educators has been addressed in a number of other international research studies. In a study conducted in Hong Kong, nursing students rated professional competence of the clinical teacher as the most important characteristic of effective teaching, followed by interpersonal relationships and the teacher's personal attributes (Nahas & Yam, 2001). According to the respondents in this study, the most important characteristics that reflect professional competence of clinical educators included being well informed, demonstrating skills, and relating theory to practice, in addition to providing feedback to students and being objective and fair. Because the study took place in Hong Kong and its results differed from the findings of other studies, which showed interpersonal relationships to be the most important characteristic, these researchers suggested that cultural differences may influence student perceptions of teaching effectiveness.

Several studies have used the Nursing Clinical Teacher Effectiveness Inventory (NCTEI) or adapted versions of the tool to investigate characteristics of "best" and "worst" clinical educators, albeit with different findings. The NCTEI was developed by Mogan and Knox (1987) and consists of five subscales: teaching ability, interpersonal relationships, personality traits, nursing competence, and evaluation. In a replication study of Mogan and Knox's work (1987), Lee, Cholowski, and Williams (2002) surveyed Australian students (N = 104) and clinical educators (N = 17) at a regional university for their perceptions of effective clinical teachers. Both the educators and the students rated interpersonal relationships as the most highly valued characteristic of effective clinical educators. Students who had limited "real-life" clinical experience valued interpersonal relationships more highly than students who had more clinical experience. While the differences were not statistically significant, the students ranked evaluation as next in importance and the educators ranked nursing competence next. A limitation of this study was the small size of the sample.

In a study of 185 Greek nursing students' and 31 clinical teachers' perceptions of the characteristics of "best" clinical instructors, interpersonal relationships were ranked first of the five NCTEI subscales by both the students and teachers, with students ranking nursing competence second and the teachers ranking it last among the subscales (Kotzabassaki et al., 1997). Using the Ideal Nursing Teacher Questionnaire, which was adapted from the NCTEI,

Johnsen, Aasgaard, Wahl, and Salminen (2002) surveyed nurse educators in Norway (N = 348) to identify their perceptions of the most important domains in educator competence. Content validity and Cronbach's alpha of the adapted tool were established. Based upon mean and confidence interval values, the nursing competence and teaching competence domains were rated as more important than evaluation skills, personality factors, and relationships with students by the Norwegian nurse educators.

Many professional nursing competencies are role modeled for students who then have a model upon which to base their own behaviors. Wiseman's (1994) study described additional role modeling behaviors including: participating in change of shift reports; asking questions about the patient's condition; reporting data to staff personnel in a timely fashion; interacting with physicians in a confident, professional manner; identifying self to patients; demonstrating caring of both patients and students; respecting patient's integrity; keeping confidential information to self; demonstrating a clean, neat appearance; providing appropriate care to patients by meeting their needs; using equipment appropriately; assisting with hands-on care when needed, and being organized in the clinical setting.

Demonstrating Professional Teaching Competence. Bergman and Gaitskill (1990) identified professional teaching competencies for the clinical nurse educator to be: planning the clinical experience and setting realistic objectives and expectations; providing useful feedback on student progress; supervising and helping students in new experiences without taking over; being objective and fair in evaluation; being flexible, and relating underlying theory to nursing practice. Having skill in high-level questioning (application, analysis, synthesis, and evaluation) was also identified as important to stimulating learning in the clinical setting (Phillips & Duke, 2001).

Krichbaum's (1994) study of the relationship of clinical teaching effectiveness and learning outcomes of baccalaureate nursing students revealed the importance of setting objectives for students in clinical rotations, providing the students with opportunities for practice as well as opportunities for observation of nurses practicing on the unit, asking effective questions, offering timely and appropriate feedback, and demonstrating enthusiasm for teaching. Krichbaum suggested that the combination of observation and practice opportunities for students in clinical settings facilitated their cognitive development as well as their "performance learning outcomes" (p. 314).

In a replication of Krichbaum's study conducted with Lebanese nursing students, Makarem, Dumit, Adra, and Kassak (2001) discovered that observing nurse-patient interactions in the clinical setting "... was positively correlated with students' ability to relate therapeutically with assigned patients and significant others" (p. 47) and act as patient advocates. They also found the clinical teacher behaviors of demonstrating flexibility, answering questions, and showing concern for the students' progress and problems, as well as the quality of discourse and specificity of feedback, to be positively and significantly correlated with achievement of learning outcomes by baccalaureate nursing students in a critical care nursing course, thus indicating effective teaching. Significant behaviors that were found to be negatively correlated with achievement of learning outcomes included quality of feedback, if the feedback was felt to be unfair or unduly critical, and the role modeling of unprofessional behaviors.

Li (1997) identified six clinical teaching behaviors rated within the top 10 most important behaviors by both students and teachers in a hospital-based training program in Hong Kong. These behaviors included: explains clearly, does not criticize the student in front of others, is a good role model, corrects students' mistakes without belittling them, is open-minded and nonjudgmental, and provides support and encouragement to students. Camiah (1998) identified important skills for new nurse clinical teachers, including educational management skills (e.g., time management, communication skills), teaching and learning skills, and professional development skills (e.g., clinical competence, academic qualifications). Effective teaching and learning skills in the clinical setting require teachers to use a variety of teaching methods, continually assess knowledge and practice skills, and provide assistance that helps students integrate theory and practice.

Fowler (1995) discussed the importance of good supervisory skills in the clinical nurse educator. These supervisory skills must be based upon knowledge, the ability to teach, and exhibiting good relationship skills. Supervisory skills have been described as "observing [students'] psychomotor skills, the[ir] ability to prioritize, and the efficiency with which [students] carry out the roles allocated to them" (Brown, Forrest & Pollock, 1998, p. 15).

Evaluative skills also emerged as having high importance for the clinical nurse educator. Evaluative skills include being able to communicate expectations clearly, demonstrate fairness in grading, provide constructive criticism, and offer new insights to students (Gignac-Caille & Oermann, 2001; Viverais-Dresler & Kutschke, 2001).

Many of the clinical teaching skills discussed in the literature are related to the educator's ability to communicate well with others. For example, Makarem et al.'s (2001) study revealed that clear communication was positively correlated with the students' ability to integrate nursing science principles into clinical decision-making and the use of the nursing process. The next section expands on the importance of developing relationships with students so that one can be effective in the role of clinical instructor.

Establishing Relationships with Students. Bergman and Gaitskill (1990) stated that clinical educator competencies for relating to students include: being realistic in expectations of students; being honest and direct; conveying confidence in and respect for the student; encouraging students to ask questions or ask for help; permitting freedom of discussion and venting of feelings, and being available to students as situations arise in the clinical setting. Beck's (1993) study revealed the perceptions of students in their first clinical experience as: feeling pervasive anxiety; feeling abandoned; encountering reality shock; envisioning self as incompetent; doubting choices, and experiencing uplifting consequences. These reactions require understanding and support from the clinical nurse educator.

Dillon and Stines (1996) conducted a phenomenological study that replicated Beck's (1991) earlier study of baccalaureate nursing students' perception of faculty caring. However, Dillon and Stines focused their study on LPN (N = 49) and nurses' aide (N = 32) students. The purpose of the study was to identify caring faculty behaviors as perceived by students. Students were asked to respond in writing with an example of what they considered to be a caring incident with faculty that they had personally experienced. The written responses were analyzed using Colaizzi's (1978) phenomenological methodology. The three themes related to faculty-student caring interactions that emerged from the analysis and illustrated faculty caring behaviors from the students' perspective were: faculty sharing and giving of themselves (e.g., spending extra time with students and providing one-on-one attention, following through, providing positive reinforcement); respecting students as unique individuals (e.g., displaying sensitivity, being perceptive of students' feelings, being friendly and calm), and role-modeling caring behaviors for students.

Whitman (1990) also identified role modeling of professional nurse behaviors in practice as a caring faculty behavior that contributes to the development of the student and teacher relationship. Other qualities that Whitman identified as important interpersonal skills include exhibiting patience, maintaining a controlled manner regardless of stress level, and collaborating with students and assisting them to become familiar with the clinical setting.

Beck's (2001) meta-analysis of the literature on caring in nursing education revealed that caring is a "process of reciprocal connection" (p. 104) as evidenced by the educator presencing (or "being there" for students), sharing, supporting, and demonstrating knowledge and competence in clinical skills. These characteristics provide students with a sense of respect and belonging, as they grow as professionals and learn to care for others. Beck suggested this leads to self-actualization for the student.

Krichbaum (1994) stated that the manner or attitude the teacher uses to convey feedback to students was important, so that students believed the teacher was concerned for their learning. Students need to have their self-esteem and self-worth validated by faculty, not feel belittled when corrected, and believe they are being respected by their faculty (Sieh & Bell, 1994). In Li's (1997) study on effective clinical behaviors in a hospital-based nursing training program, the following behaviors emerged as being important to establishing a positive relationship with students: not criticizing a student in front of others; not belittling students; explaining clearly, and being open-minded and nonjudgmental.

If the clinical nurse educator is to prepare nurses who think and who exemplify curiosity, skepticism, and courage (Reich, 1991), and who are able to practice in a variety of environments, then the role in the practice setting is to be "coach, counselor and facilitator of discussion" (Rossignol, 2000, p. 245). Rossignol asserted that utilizing these roles in the clinical arena actively engages students in the learning process. While the use of pre- or post-conferences is valuable for students to learn from their peers and vent their anxieties and frustration, Rossignol also stated that clinical post-conferences should provide an opportunity for dialogue in a "co-operative student-faculty partnership" (p. 249) that facilitates development of the learner's higher-level thinking.

Using Personal Attributes to Facilitate Learning. In addition to being able to develop relationships with students, other personal attributes that are believed to facilitate learning have been identified by Bergman and Gaitskill (1990). Personal attributes that facilitate learning and are important for clinical teachers to possess to be effective in their roles are: showing enthusiasm for teaching and nursing; demonstrating self-control; being cooperative and patient; displaying flexibility when needed; admitting to limitations and mistakes honestly; displaying a sense of humor, and possessing good communication skills. Among the communication skills that are important for effective clinical teaching are establishing practitioner's role expectations of the teacher and negotiating students' learning experiences with practitioners (Davies, White, Riley, & Twinn, 1996).

As a result of her study, Krichbaum (1994) described the following personal characteristics needed for the effective clinical nurse educator: having a positive attitude; showing a willingness to discuss what one knows, what one believes, and how one practices; having a sense of one's own strengths and weaknesses, and possessing self-confidence. While Bergman and Gaitskill's (1990) study did not rate humor as particularly important, Nahas' (1998) study of humor as used in clinical settings with undergraduate nursing students in Australia did. Having a sense of humor and being able to make people laugh is "part of human behaviour"(p. 664) and it is a language that is universal, acting as a means of communication to transcend differences and illuminate similarities (Johnston, 1990, cited in Nahas, 1998). Nahas demonstrated that humor could alleviate anxiety and stress for nursing students, and it could enhance learning by enabling the student to gain control in a stressful situation. The themes that emerged from this phenomenological study indicated that, with the use of humor and laughter, the clinical teacher is identified as being human, genuine, able to create a positive clinical environment that facilitates learning, and connecting with students. The caveat is that the teacher must be aware of the personal nature of humor, understanding that it can be destructive and must never be used against students. Ulloth's (2003) qualitative study on the use of humor in undergraduate nursing education, while not focused on clinical teaching, supported Nahas' findings that humor can facilitate student learning, make learning fun, and strengthen student/faculty relationships.

Role of the Preceptor

For the purposes of this monograph, "preceptor" is used to describe a nonfaculty registered nurse or other health care provider who works with nursing students, in a close one-on-one relationship, in a clinical setting, for a specified period of time. The key aspect of this role is that it is a collaborative relationship, established through mutual agreement between faculty from an educational institution and practicing clinicians in hospitals or health care agencies in order to provide on-site supervision and clinical instruction to students. "Preceptees" may be students enrolled in undergraduate programs preparing for initial licensure, or they may be enrolled in graduate programs preparing for advanced practice. In general, at the undergraduate level, the preceptor model has been used with students who are nearing completion of their educational programs. Preceptorships may also be used to orient new graduates to their first position or to orient registered nurses to clinical specialty areas. Although preceptors are not usually faculty per se, they serve a vital role in the education of nurses at all levels. The effectiveness of the preceptors' role performance and, ultimately the success of the students with whom they work, is influenced by the nurse educator who coordinates the preceptorship and collaborates with the preceptor.

Research literature related to the preceptor role is organized around the following themes: description of preceptor functions and characteristics; benefits and difficulties associated with the preceptor model of education; and faculty roles and responsibilities related to working with preceptors.

Functioning as a Preceptor. As experienced and competent clinicians, preceptors serve as role models and resource persons who help students develop confidence and competence and socialize them into the nursing profession (Letizia & Jennrich, 1998; Greene & Puetzer, 2002). O'Malley et al. (2000) suggested that preceptorships ease the transition from learner to clinician and limit "reality shock" for new graduates. Ferguson and Calder (1993) demonstrated increased levels of self-confidence and role socialization among undergraduate nursing students who participated in preceptorships.

In a study examining desirable preceptor characteristics among Army Nurse Corps preceptors, Bartz and Srsic-Stoehr (1994) reported that preceptees indicated that "clinical competence" was the most important characteristic of an effective preceptor. Similarly, in Coates and Gormley's (1997) mixed method study of preceptorships at one university in the United Kingdom, knowledge of the clinical area and clinical experience were identified by students, preceptors, nurse teachers, and managers as the preceptors' greatest role assets; lack of adequate time to teach students was a barrier. Recommendations from this study included developing more clarity around the expectations of the preceptor role and providing an adequate orientation program for preceptors.

Using an adapted version of the Invitational Teaching Survey instrument to identify desirable preceptor characteristics as perceived by perioperative nurses (N = 57) who had experienced a recent preceptoring relationship, Finger and Pape (2002) reported that demonstrating current knowledge, encouraging self-confidence, being professional and efficient, and being friendly ranked high as desirable preceptor characteristics. Interestingly, the characteristic that received the single highest mean score in this study was learning the preceptees' names. The reliability of the revised tool and its subscales was established using Cronbach's alpha correlation coefficient and deemed acceptable. Other preceptor functions described in the literature include coaching, developing skills, fostering independence, assessing performance, promoting socialization into the profession, developing confidence and competence, and empowering students by including them in the preceptor's daily work responsibilities (Oermann, 1996; Daigle, 2001; Ohrling & Hallberg, 2001; Hrobsky & Kersbergen, 2002).

Some researchers have investigated the preceptor role from the perspective of the preceptor. Ohrling and Hallberg (2001) used phenomenological-hermeneutic interpretation to investigate the meaning of preceptorship as experienced by nurse preceptors in Sweden. The seventeen nurses who participated in this study were preceptors to undergraduate nursing students in their last year of education. Two themes emerged from the preceptors' narratives about what it meant to be a preceptor – facilitating student learning with patient care and sheltering students during the learning process, which was related to negotiating learning experiences for the student.

In another qualitative study, Hrobsky and Kersbergen (2002) investigated preceptors' feelings when involved with undergraduate students who performed unsatisfactorily in the clinical setting. Preceptors in this study reported feeling a sense of self-doubt, fear, and anxiety about reporting observations to faculty that would lead to a student's failure. Both of these studies illustrate the responsibility for student learning that preceptors feel in their role and the need for preparation to effectively assume the role.

Several researchers examined effective characteristics that influence the preceptor-student relationship, and a majority of them found that the more open and supportive the preceptor, the better the learning experience for the student. Hayes (2001), in a study with nurse practitioner students, found that an open supportive approach by the preceptor, which they termed a "humanistic precepting style" may be just as important as clinical expertise and that the "tone" of the clinical setting can either facilitate or hinder the learning process. Likewise, Myrick and Yonge (2001) found that "when preceptors genuinely support and work with students in the practice setting and the staff accepts them as part of the team, a climate that is conducive to learning and critical thinking is established" (p. 461). In a study conducted in China, Chang, Liao, Dou, and Hu (2000) found a significant positive correlation ($p < .01$) between scores for professional competence, teaching competence, interpersonal relationships, and personality characteristics of preceptors for nursing administration students.

Benefits and Challenges of the Preceptor Model. Benefits of the preceptor model are well documented in both research and nonresearch nursing literature. Among the most commonly cited benefits of the preceptor model are an improved learning environment for students through the creation of clinical learning partnerships, enhanced clinical skills, increased competence of graduates, and the integration and enactment of the professional role (Stevenson, Doorley, Moddeman, & Benson-Landau, 1995; Byrd, Hood, & Youtsey, 1997; Johnson, 1999; Gibson & Hauri, 2000; Kaviani & Stillwell, 2000).

In a phenomenological study that triangulated data obtained from interviews with students, preceptors, and faculty, Nehls, Rather, and Guyette (1997) identified learning "nursing thinking" (p. 222) and "concernful attention" (or caring) (p. 225) as major benefits of the preceptor experience. Preceptors helped students learn how to see the big picture in clinical situations. In the words of these authors, "preceptors taught by example that caring leads nurses to notice problems, consider relevant data, and decide which interventions are most likely to be effective" (Nehls et al., p. 255).

For preceptors, the benefits identified have included personal and professional development and increased job satisfaction (Stevenson et al., 1995; Kaviani & Stillwell, 2000). In a survey of 295 preceptors, Yonge, Krahn, Trojan, and Reid (1997) identified exposure to new knowledge, which they viewed as a form of continuing education, as an additional advantage to preceptors. Benefits to the profession as a whole have also been described. These benefits include development of collaborative collegial relationships between nurse educators and nurse practitioners and reciprocal development of the preceptors' and faculty members' knowledge (Johnson, 1999; Kaviani & Stillwell, 2000; Ohrling & Hallberg, 2001). Well-prepared nursing graduates who are able to function effectively affect the entire profession and ultimately, patient care outcomes.

For clinical agencies, effective preceptorships may also enhance recruitment and retention of staff. Matthews and Nunley (1992) reported that orientation programs that offer a positive experience (i.e., where new employees feel welcomed and are included in orientation goal-setting) have been shown to reduce turnover rates by as much as 35%.

Although numerous studies have demonstrated a positive impact on the individual nurse and ultimately the nursing profession, using the preceptor model of education also carries additional responsibilities and workload requirements for individual preceptors and faculty. A principal difficulty that has been identified as impacting preceptors is lack of time to effectively perform the role (Coates & Gormley, 1997; Pfeil, 1999; Kaviani & Stillwell, 2000; Allen & Simpson, 2000; Hayes, 2001; Lyon & Peach, 2001). This lack of time has been attributed to a variety of factors, the most prominent being the need to increase efficiency and productivity in the current health care climate.

Another identified challenge to the preceptor model relates to preceptors' lack of comfort with the role itself. Numerous studies have cited the need for preceptor training programs and several studies have examined the perceptions of preceptors before and after orientation to the role. Laforet-Fliesser, Ward-Griffin, and Beynon (1999), who studied baccalaureate students in a community setting, found that preceptors were comfortable with providing feedback and with encouraging students to use agency personnel for advice, but they were less confident with selecting learning experiences congruent with course objectives and with trusting the students' readiness to work with communities. Similarly, Pfeil (1999) found that learning objectives needed to be made relevant for preceptors. Subjects in Allen and Simpson's (2000) study indicated that they felt they were inadequately prepared to be preceptors and that support for precepting did not meet their expectations. These subjects also indicated that they felt their role was neither valued nor adequately acknowledged by teachers, students, or managers. Other studies (Usher, Nolan, Reser, Owens, & Tollefson, 1999; Kaviani & Stillwell, 2000) also cited the need for more formal recognition of the preceptor role in clinical practice.

A final area of challenge with using preceptors is the attitude of the preceptors themselves. Daigle (2001) expressed concern regarding the use of preceptors "whose attitude is jaded" (p. 4) and how, despite good clinical skills, such an attitude can negatively impact the outcome of the preceptor experience. In contrast, Nehls et al. (1997) demonstrated that preceptors who modeled an attitude of caring in patient care and a concern for the learner positively impacted outcomes of the preceptor experience.

Faculty Roles and Responsibilities. Studies examining faculty roles in using the preceptor model of education have identified several specific responsibilities. These responsibilities include: building alliances; orienting students and preceptors; maintaining open communication; sharing responsibility for evaluation of learning, and providing support to and recognition of individual preceptors.

One faculty responsibility is the orientation of preceptors to the role. Several studies reported the benefits of preceptor orientation programs and gave examples of specific content to be included in those programs (Byrd, Hood, & Youtsey, 1997; Yonge et al., 1997; Laforet-Fliesser et al., 1999; O'Malley et al., 2000; Trevitt, Grealish, & Reaby, 2001; Myrick & Yonge, 2001). The importance of assessing the skills and attitudes of both students and preceptors before clinical placement, as well as the need for faculty to take an active role in preceptor orientation, was emphasized by Yonge et al. (1997) and Letizia and Jennrich (1998).

Phillips and Duke (2001) described the need to teach preceptors how to ask high-level questions. The findings of their study, which was conducted in Australia and used a comparative descriptive design, indicated that clinical teachers typically asked more questions generally as well as higher-level questions than did preceptors. Using the Chi-square, the difference was statistically significant between the two groups ($p < .0001$). The need to include examples of how to use effective pedagogical strategies in preceptor orientation programs was discussed by

Ohrling and Hallberg (2001). Westra and Graziano (1992) used a comparative study to examine perceived needs of preceptors before and after a formal preceptor orientation program. They found a significant difference in preceptors' perceptions of their need for more information related to evaluating novice performances (p <.03) following the formal orientation program.

Trevitt et al. (2001) described the development, implementation, and evaluation of a "self-directed" preceptorship orientation program with modules for preceptors and preceptees. Using qualitative evaluation measures (i.e., focus groups), these researchers found that the self-directed format strengthened the preceptorship because it reinforced principles of learning and communication techniques and clarified expectations for both students and preceptors.

Maintaining open communication with and providing faculty support to preceptors ensures positive outcomes. Using a descriptive, correlational design, Dibert and Goldenberg (1995) examined nurse preceptors' (N = 116) perceptions of benefits, support, and commitment to the preceptor role. They found that preceptors' commitment to their role was significantly (p < .05) and positively correlated to their perception of support, benefits, and the frequency with which they served as preceptors. Usher et al. (1999) replicated that study and reported similar results. Ferguson (1995), DeLong and Bechtel (1999) and Gibson and Hauri (2000) documented preceptors' need or desire for faculty support and feedback and found that although there were differences in the level of support required by individual preceptors, in general they desired assistance with evaluating student learning. As Hrobsky and Kersberngen (2002) indicated, the need for faculty support is likely to be greater when students are not performing well. They recommended that "listening, being supportive, and following up after the experience enhances the collaborative relationship…and facilitates preceptors' coping with clinical performance failure" (p. 553). Lyon and Peach (2001) also found that good communication with faculty was a major factor in determining whether preceptors were willing to continue serving in that role.

In a study using grounded theory methodology, Myrick (2002) found that preceptees' ability to think critically was directly affected by staff acceptance and that certain preceptor behaviors (e.g., role modeling and priority-setting) also contributed to the preceptees' developing critical thinking skills. In addition, similar to Phillips and Duke (2001), Myrick found that preceptors tended to ask more low-level rather than high-level questions and suggested that faculty seek ways to work with preceptors to improve questioning techniques and thereby enhance critical thinking.

Finally, the need for recognition of preceptors has been well documented. Kaviani and Stillwell (2000) cited the need for formal recognition of the preceptor role in clinical practice and Usher et al. (1999) pointed out that support and recognition by the institution and the preceptor's co-workers is vital. Similarly, Ohrling and Hallberg (2001) made suggestions for increasing awareness of the value of preceptors in nursing practice. Allen (2002) studied preceptors in a mental health setting. While many of the preceptors interviewed for that study described a sense of reward gained from watching the students' progress, others indicated a desire for acknowledgment and recognition or other tangible rewards. Hayes (1994) and Lyon and Peach (2001) also emphasized the importance of understanding and acknowledging the increasing pressures and time limitations that many preceptors face.

Within nursing education, the use of preceptorships has been demonstrated to be a valuable tool for facilitating learning and learner development as well as fostering role transition for students and new graduates. However, careful selection and orientation of preceptors, along with faculty support and institutional valuing of those who assume the preceptor role, is critical to ensure positive learning experiences and achievement of desired learning outcomes for preceptees, as well as personal satisfaction and professional growth for preceptors. Preceptorships hold tremendous potential for enhancing learner development, but they also require a concomitant commitment of faculty time and effort.

Identified Gaps in the Literature

The variety of articles reviewed enhances understanding of the knowledge, skills, and attitudes nurse educators need to facilitate student learning. However, areas can be identified where ongoing knowledge development related to facilitating learning is essential for advancing the science of nursing education. The following areas reflecting how the science of nursing education can be further developed were gleaned from specific recommendations by authors as well as by identifying "gaps" in the review of the recent research literature. Many of the gaps appeared in the area of clinical teaching.

There is little in the literature referring to clinical teaching in graduate education, although a few studies do reflect the use of preceptors in preparing students for advanced practice roles. Although preceptors are commonly used in nursing programs, including those in teaching and administration, the ways in which preceptors are prepared, utilized, and their competency evaluated, particularly at the graduate level, are not adequately addressed in the literature. Most of the research literature regarding the faculty role in working with preceptors was descriptive in nature. With the shortage of qualified faculty and a possible increase in the use of preceptors for clinical supervision of nursing students at all levels, there is need for more empirical data on the most effective roles for faculty in this model of clinical teaching. There is also a need for research on how nurse educators develop and maintain effective collegial relationships with nurses in clinical settings to create the most positive learning environments for students and staff (Owen, 1993).

This review did not reveal any studies related to the significance of the sociocultural context within which clinical teaching in nursing occurs. There were some indications that the sociocultural context affects how students respond and learn in the clinical setting. With the increasing diversity of patients, students, faculty and health care workers, this is an area that deserves further attention. In addition, most of the literature that was reviewed addressed clinical teaching in acute care settings. No studies were found regarding clinical teaching competencies in non-acute care settings such as homes, day care centers, rehabilitation centers, long-term care facilities, hospices, schools, clinics, or community and public health settings. Similarly, studies about teaching in the mental health arena were lacking. These settings may require different skills and knowledge to effectively facilitate learning. If more health care services are being provided in non-acute care settings and curricula are increasingly including courses with learning experiences provided in community health settings, we need to know what clinical teaching competencies are needed by educators in such settings.

Few studies were found on how to effectively use the clinical pre- and post- conference time to facilitate student learning. This is a time when effective discourse can guide students to interpret the meaning and significance of the clinical situations they encounter; reflective, situated understanding of practice situations can occur; and student learning can be enhanced. Further study of how to design clinical learning activities that best use this time with students is warranted.

Based on some of the literature reviewed, there appears to be a gap in the knowledge and competence of nurse educators in relation to leadership and advocacy, health care economics, health information systems, and health systems management. This has the potential of impeding educators' ability to facilitate student learning in these areas. Similarly, there was little in the literature regarding educators' understanding of ethical development and facilitating student learning in this area. Hamric (2001) pointed out the importance of ethical development in clinical faculty, because it is the clinical teacher, typically in post-conference, who encourages analysis of ethical dilemmas and application of ethical knowledge to clinical experiences. Educator competencies required to effectively cover this area need to be explicated.

The literature does not adequately address the perceived theory-practice gap so often identified by educators and the skills that are needed by educators to bridge it. The challenge of maintaining clinical competence while primarily working in an academic setting is frequently identified as a source of role strain for educators. How work-related stress might affect the facilitation of student learning was addressed in only one article by Oermann (1998), who focused on clinical teachers. Given the nursing shortage and exodus or retirement of faculty and practitioners from the profession, this would appear to be a markedly understudied topic.

Harris (1998), conducting an integrative review of the literature in higher education, concluded that there was little research on the characteristics of ineffective teachers, or on how one becomes an effective teacher. However, Young and Shaw (1999) did report ratings of ineffective teachers in their survey of students, and some unpublished dissertation research has begun to address the "how" question. Much of the published research reviewed summarized characteristics of effective teachers, with less discussion of how to develop these characteristics. The literature does not really inform the nurse educator how to develop the skills identified as important to be effective teachers in the classroom and in clinical settings in order to facilitate student learning. In addition, much of the research literature related to facilitating learning has been conducted with undergraduate education and students; graduate education and students have received less attention.

Priorities for Future Research

Both quantitative and qualitative approaches are needed to further understand nurse educator competencies related to facilitating student learning. In addition, large, multisite studies conducted in a variety of academic and health care settings would contribute to developing the science of nursing education in this area. The following questions reflect priorities for future research:

- What knowledge, skills, and attitudes are needed for effective teaching in master's and doctoral nursing programs?

- What knowledge, skills, and attitudes among educators and preceptors best facilitate student learning in both undergraduate and graduate level programs when clinical preceptor models are used? What are the most effective ways to develop the requisite knowledge, skills, and attitudes in educators and preceptors to most effectively use the clinical preceptor model?

- How can educators collaborate most effectively with practitioners to facilitate student learning in the clinical setting?

- What knowledge, skills, and attitudes do educators need to use teaching methodologies that respect the sociocultural context within which learning occurs in clinical and classroom settings?

- How do educators become effective teachers and achieve competence in facilitating learning? What evidence-based indicators can be used to measure the extent of the nurse educator's competence? What experiences most profoundly shape the educator's developing competence in facilitating learning?

- What specific instructional strategies increase the effectiveness of clinical teaching?

- What instructional strategies enhance the use of pre- and post-conferences as a clinical teaching tool?

- What qualitative and quantitative measures and methods are most useful for evaluating teacher effectiveness?

- How does the use of distance education affect the acquisition of the social and behavioral skills demanded in the nursing profession? Can these skills be effectively acquired through the use of distance learning?

- What are best practices to facilitate student learning in nursing education so that they can provide quality care in a rapidly changing health care environment?

References

Adams, K.A. (2002). *What colleges and universities want in new faculty.* Washington, DC: Association of American Colleges and Universities.

Allen, C. (2002). Peers and partners: A stakeholders evaluation of preceptorships in mental health nursing. *Nurse Researcher, 9*(3), 68.

Allen, C., & Simpson, A. (2000). Peers and partners: Working together to strengthen preceptorships in mental health nursing. *Journal of Psychiatric & Mental Health Nursing, 7*(6), 505-514.

American Association of Colleges of Nursing. (2000). AACN white paper: Distance technology in nursing education: Assessing a new frontier. *Journal of Professional Nursing, 16*(2),116-122.

Austin, S.I. (1999). Baccalaureate nursing faculty performance of nursing computer literacy skills and curriculum integration of these skills through teaching practice. *Journal of Nursing Education, 38*(6), 260-266.

Bartz, C., & Srsic-Stoehr, K.M. (1994). Nurses' views on preceptorship programs and preceptor and preceptee experiences. Army Nurse Preceptorship Program. *Journal of Nursing Staff Development, 10*(13), 153-158.

Beck, C. T. (1991). How students perceive faculty caring: A phenomenological study. *Nurse Educator, 16*(5), 18-22.

Beck, C. T. (1993). Nursing students' initial clinical experience: A phenomenological study. *International Journal of Nursing Studies, 30*(6), 489-497.

Beck, C. T. (2001). Caring within nursing education: A metasynthesis. *Journal of Nursing Education, 40*(3), 101-109.

Beeson, S.A., & Kring, D.L. (1999). The effects of two teaching methods on nursing students' factual knowledge and performance of psychomotor skills. *Journal of Nursing Education, 38*(7), 357-359.

Benor, D. E., & Leviyof, I. (1997). The development of student's perceptions of effective teaching: The ideal, best and poorest clinical teacher in nursing. *Journal of Nursing Education, 36*(5), 206-211.

Bergman, K., & Gaitskill, T. (1990). Faculty and student perceptions of effective clinical teachers. *Journal of Professional Nursing, 6*(1), 33-44.

Billings, D. (1995). Preparing nursing faculty for information-age teaching and learning. *Computers in Nursing, 13*(6), 268-270.

Boyer, E. (1990). *Scholarship reconsidered: Priorities of the professoriate* (Report No. ISBN-0-931050-43-X). Princeton, NJ: Carnegie Foundation for the Advancement of Teaching. (ERIC Document Reproduction Service No. ED 326 149)

Brown, N., Forrest, S., & Pollock, L. C. (1998). The ideal role of the nurse teacher in the clinical area: A comparison of the perspectives of mental health, learning difficulties and general nurses. *Journal of Psychiatric and Mental Health Nursing, 5*(1), 11-19.

Byrd, C.Y., Hood, L. & Youtsey, N. (1997). Student and preceptor perceptions of factors in a successful learning partnership. *Journal of Professional Nursing, 13*(16), 344-351.

Camiah, S. (1998). New skills required of nurse tutors in the UK: A study within two Project 2000 pilot schemes for pre-registration nursing courses. *Nurse Education Today, 18*(2), 93-100.

Campbell, J. (1997). Perspectives of distinguished teaching award winners: Personal meanings of teaching (Doctoral dissertation, University of Massachusetts, Amherst, 1997). *Dissertation Abstracts International, 58,* 394.

Chang, C., Liao, M., Dou, S., & Hu, S. (2000). An evaluation of preceptors in nursing administration practice. *Journal of Nursing* (China), *47*(6), 32-42.

Chickering, A., & Gamson, Z. (1987). Seven principles for good practice in undergraduate education. *American Association of Higher Education Bulletin, 39*(7), 3-7.

Clarke, B., & James, C. (1993). The knowledge base for teaching and facilitating. The teacher as a learner. *Nurse Times, 89*(46), i-viii.

Coates, V.E., & Gormley, E. (1997). Learning the practice of nursing: Views about preceptorship. *Nurse Education Today, 17*(2), 91-98.

Colazzi, P. (1978). Psychological research as the phenomenologist views it. In R. S. Valle & M. King (Eds)., *Existential-phenomenological alternatives for psychology,* (pp. 48-71). New York: Oxford University Press.

Cobb, K. L. & Billings, D. M. (2000). Assessing distance education programs in nursing. In: J. Novotny (Ed.), *Distance education in nursing* (pp. 85-112). New York: Springer.

Daigle, J. (2001). Preceptors in nursing education–facilitating student learning. *Kansas Nurse, 76*(4), 3-6.

Davies, S., White, E., Riley, E. & Twinn, S. (1996). How can nurse teachers be more effective in practice settings? *Nurse Education Today, 16*(1), 19-27.

De Grave, W.S., Dolmans, D., & van der Vleuten, C. (1999). Profiles of effective tutors in problem-based learning: Scaffolding student learning. *Medical Education, 33*(12), 901-906.

DeLong, T.H., & Bechtel, G.A. (1999). Enhancing relationships between nursing faculty and clinical preceptors. *Journal for Nurses in Staff Development, 15*(4), 148-151.

DeNeef, A.L. (2002). *The Preparing Future Faculty Program: What difference does it make?* Washington, DC: Association of American Colleges and Universities.

Dibert, C., & Goldenberg, D. (1995). Preceptors' perceptions of benefits, rewards, supports and commitment to the preceptor role. *Journal of Advanced Nursing, 21*(6), 1144-1151.

Diekelmann, N. (2001). Narrative pedagogy: Heideggerian hermeneutical analyses of lived Experiences of students, teachers, and clinicians. *Advances in Nursing Science, 23*(3), 53-71.

Dillon, R. S., & Stines, P. W. (1996). A phenomenological study of faculty-student caring interactions. *Journal of Nursing Education, 35*(3), 113-118.

Ferguson, L.M. (1995). Faculty support for nurse preceptors. *Nursing Connections, 8*(2), 37-49.

Ferguson, L., & Calder, B., (1993). A comparison of preceptor and educator valuing of nursing student clinical performance criteria. *Journal of Nursing Education, 32*(1), 30-36.

Finger, S. D., & Pape, T. M. (2002). Invitational theory and perioperative nursing preceptorships. *Association of Operating Room Nurses (AORN) Journal, 76*(4), 630.

Fowler, J. (1995). Nurse's perceptions of the elements of good supervision. *Nursing Times, 91*(22), 33-37.

Gibson, S.E., & Hauri, C. (2000). The pleasure of your company: Attitudes and opinions of preceptors toward nurse practitioner preceptees. *Journal of the American Academy of Nursing Practitioners, 12*(9), 360-363.

Gignac-Caille A. M., & Oermann, M. H. (2001). Student and faculty perceptions of effective clinical instructors in ADN programs. *Journal of Nursing Education, 40*(8), 347-353.

Goorapah, D. (1997). Clinical competence/clinical credibility. *Nurse Education Today, 17*(4), 297-302.

Greene, M.T., & Puetzer, M. (2002). The value of mentoring: A strategic approach to retention and recruitment. *Journal of Nursing Care Quality, 17*(1), 63-70.

Hamric, A. B. (2001). Ethics development for clinical faculty. *Nursing Outlook, 49*(3), 115-117.

Harris, A. (1998). Effective teaching: A review of literature. *School Leadership and Management, 18*(2), 169-183.

Hayes, E. (1994). Helping preceptors mentor the next generation of nurse practitioners. *Nurse Practitioner, 19*(6), 62-65

Hayes, E.F. (2001). Factors that facilitate or hinder mentoring in the nurse practitioner preceptor/ student relationship. *Clinical Excellence for Nurse Practitioners, 5*(2), 111-118.

Hewlett, P.O. (1993). The relationship between selected variables and self-perceived competencies as an adult educator among nursing faculties in RN to BSN completion programs (Doctoral dissertation, The University of Mississippi, 1993). *Dissertation Abstracts International.* (UMI No. PUZ93261)

Hill, F.A. (1995). Characteristics of exemplary university professors as perceived by master's degree students at Northern Arizona University (Doctoral dissertation, Northern Arizona University, 1995). *Dissertation Abstracts International, 56*, 1739.

Hrobsky, P.E. & Kersbergen, A.L. (2002). Preceptors' perceptions of clinical performance failure. *Journal of Nursing Education, 41*(12), 550-554.

Jackson, D., & Sullivan, J.R. (1999). Integrating the creative arts into a midwifery curriculum: A teaching innovation report. *Nurse Education Today, 19*(7), 527-532.

Johnsen, K. O., Aasgaard, H. S., Wahl, A. K., & Salminen, L. (2002). Nurse educator competence: A study of Norwegian nurse educators' opinions of the importance and application of different nurse educator competence domains. *Journal of Nursing Education, 41*(7), 295-301.

Johnson, C.G. (1999). Evaluating preceptorship in a distance nursing program. *Journal of National Black Nurses Association, 10*(2), 65-78.

Johnston, A.K., & Tinning, R.S. (2001). Meeting the challenge of problem-based learning: Developing the facilitators. *Nurse Education Today, 21*(3) 161-169.

Johnston, R. (1990). Humour: A preventive health strategy. *International Journal for the Advancement of Counselling, 13*(3), 257-265.

Kaiser, C.R. (2000). A study of the attributes of effective teachers in an accelerated business program (Doctoral dissertation, University of Wisconsin, Madison, 2002). *Dissertation Abstracts International, A-61*, 1710.

Kaviani, N., & Stillwell, Y. (2000). An evaluative study of clinical preceptorship, *Nurse Education Today, 20*(3), 218-226.

Kelly, C.M. (2002). Investing in the future of nursing education. *Nursing Education Perspectives, 23*(1), 24-29.

Knight, C. (2001).The skills of teaching social work practice in the generalist/foundation curriculum: BSW and MSW student views. *Journal of Social Work Education, 37*(3), 507-521.

Kotzabassaki, S., Panou, M., Dimou, F., Karabagli, A., Koutsopoulou, B., & Ikonomou, U. (1997). Nursing students' and faculty's perceptions of the characteristics of "best" and "worst" clinical teachers: A replication study. *Journal of Advanced Nursing, 26*(4), 817-824.

Krichbaum, K. K. (1994). Clinical teaching effectiveness described in relation to learning outcomes of baccalaureate nursing students. *Journal of Nursing Education, 33*(7), 306-316.

Laforet-Fliesser, Y., Ward-Griffin, C. & Beynon, C. (1999). Self-efficacy of preceptors in the community: A partnership between service and education. *Nurse Education Today, 19*(1), 41-52.

Lee, W., Cholowski, K., & Williams, A. K. (2002). Nursing students' and clinical educators' perceptions of characteristics of effective clinical educators in an Australian university school of nursing. *Journal of Advanced Nursing, 39*(5), 412-420.

Letizia, M. & Jennrich, J. (1998). A review of preceptorship in undergraduate nursing education: Implications for staff development. *The Journal of Continuing Education in Nursing, 29*(5), 211-216.

Li, M. (1997). Perceptions of effective clinical teaching behaviors in a hospital-based nurse training program. *Journal of Advanced Nursing, 26*(6), 1252-1261.

Link, D.G., & Scholtz, S.M. (2000). Educational technology and the faculty role: What you don't know can hurt you. *Nurse Educator, 25*(6), 274-276.

Lowman, J. (1995). *What constitutes masterful teaching. Mastering the techniques of teaching.* San Francisco: Jossey-Bass.

Lyon, D.E., & Peach, J. (2001). Primary care providers' views of precepting nurse practitioner students. *Journal of the American Academy of Nurse Practitioners, 13*(5), 237-240.

Makarem, S., Dumit, N. Y., Adra, M., & Kassak, K. (2001). Teaching effectiveness and learning outcomes of baccalaureate nursing students in a critical care practicum: A Lebanese experience. *Nursing Outlook, 49*(1), 43-49.

Marashio, P. (1995). Designing questions to help students peel back the layers of a text. *Interdisciplinary Humanities, 12*(1), 27-31,

Mathews, J.J., & Nunley, C. (1992). Rejuvenating orientation to increase nurse satisfaction and retention. *Journal of Staff Development, 8*(4), 159-164.

McNeil, B., Elfrink, V. L., Bickford, C. J., Pierce, S. T., Beyea, S. C., Averill, C., & Klappenbach, C. (2003). Nursing information technology knowledge, skills, and preparation of student nurses, nursing faculty, and clinicians: A U. S. survey. *Journal of Nursing Education, 42*(8), 341-349.

Mhaolrunaigh, S.N., & Clifford, C. (1998). The preparation of teachers for shared learning environments. *Nurse Education Today, 18*(3), 178-182.

Milstead, J., & Nelson, R. (1998). Preparation for an online asynchronous university doctoral course: Lessons learned. *Computers in Nursing, 16*(5), 247-258.

Mogan, J., & Knox, J. E. (1987). Characteristics of "best" and "worst" clinical teachers as perceived by university nursing faculty and students. *Journal of Advanced Nursing, 12*(3), 331-337.

Murphy, S.A., Scott, C.S., & Mandel, L.P. (1996). Clinical knowledge and skill priorities in substance abuse education: A nursing faculty longitudinal survey. *Journal of Nursing Education, 35*(8), 356-360.

Myrick, F. (2002). Preceptorship and critical thinking in nursing education. *Journal of Nursing Education, 41*(4), 154

Myrick, F. & Yonge, O.J. (2001). Creating a climate for critical thinking in the preceptorship experience. *Nursing Education Today, 21*(6), 461-467.

Nahas, V. L. (1998). Humour: A phenomenological study within the context of clinical education. *Nurse Education Today, 18*(8), 663-672.

Nahas, V. L., Nour, V., & Al-Nobani, M. (1999). Jordanian undergraduate nursing student's perceptions of effective clinical teachers. *Nurse Education Today, 19*(8), 639-648.

Nahas, V.L., & Yam, B.M. (2001). Hong Kong nursing students' perceptions of effective clinical teachers. *Journal of Nursing Education, 40*(5), 233-237.

Nehls, N., Rather, M. & Guyette, M. (1997). The preceptor model of clinical instruction: The lived experience of students, preceptors, and faculty-of-record. *Journal of Nursing Education, 36*(5), 220-231.

Nesler, M. S., Hanner, M. B., Melburg,V., & McGowan, S. (2001). Professional socialization of baccalaureate nursing students: Can students in distance nursing programs become socialized? *Journal of Nursing Education,40*(7), 293-302.

Nosek, C. (2003). Going online: The lived experience of students and teachers in undergraduate nursing education. Unpublished doctoral dissertation, University of Wisconsin, Madison. UMI No. AAI308969.

Oermann, M. H. (1996). A study of preceptor roles in clinical teaching. *Nursing Connections, 9*(4), 57-64.

Oermann, M. H. (1998). Work-related stress of clinical nursing faculty. *Journal of Nursing Education, 37*(7), 302-304.

Ohrling, K., & Hallberg, I.R. (2001). The meaning of preceptorship: Nurses' lived experience of being a preceptor. *Journal of Advanced Nursing, 33*(4), 530-540.

O'Malley, C., Cunliffe, E., Hunter, S., & Breeze, J., (2000). Preceptorship in practice. *Nursing Standard, 14*(28), 45.

Owen, S. (1993). A multidimensional role for nurse teachers in the clinical area. *Journal of Clinical Nursing, 2*(1), 53-54.

Pfeil, M. (1999). Preceptorship: The progression from student to staff nurse. *Journal of Child Health Care, 3*(3), 13-18.

Phillips, N., & Duke, M. (2001). The questioning skills of clinical teachers and preceptors: A comparative study. *Journal of Advanced Nursing, 33*(4), 523-529.

Pinsky, L.E., & Irby, D.M. (1997). If at first you don't succeed: Using failure to improve teaching. *Academic Medicine, 72*(11), 973-976.

Preston-Whyte, M.E., Clark, R., Petersen, S., & Fraser, R.C. (1999). The views of academic and clinical teachers in Leicester Medical School on criteria to assess teaching competence in the small-group setting. *Medical Teacher, 21*(5), 500-505.

Reich, R. (1991). *The work of nations: Preparing ourselves for 21ˢᵗ century capitalism.* New York: Knopf.

Rossignol, M. (2000). Verbal and cognitive activities between and among students and faculty in clinical conferences. *Journal of Nursing Education, 39*(6), 245-250.

Saranto, K., & Tallberg, M. (1998). Nursing informatics in nursing education: A challenge to nurse teachers. *Nurse Education Today, 18*(1), 79-87.

Sherman, R. C. (1998). Using the World Wide Web to teach everyday applications of social psychology. *Teaching of Psychology, 25*(3), 212-216.

Shoultz, J., & Amundson, M.J. (1998). Nurse educators' knowledge of primary health care: Implications for community-based education, practice, and research. *Nursing and Health Care Perspectives, 19*(3), 114-119.

Sieh, S., & Bell, S. K. (1994). Perceptions of effective clinical teachers in associated degree programs. *Journal of Nursing Education, 33*(9), 389-394.

Stevenson, B., Doorley, J., Moddeman, G., & Benson-Landau, M. (1995). The preceptor experience: A qualitative study of perceptions of nurse preceptors regarding the preceptor role. *Journal of Nursing Staff Development, 11*(3), 160-165.

Tang, T.L. (1997). Teaching evaluation at a public institution of higher education: Factors related to the overall teaching effectiveness. *Public Personnel Management, 26*(3), 379-389.

Thach, E.C., & Murphy, K.L. (1995). Competencies for distance education professionals. *Educational Technology Research Development, 43*(1), 57-79.

Thomas, B. (1992). Challenges for teachers of women's health. *Nurse Educator, 17*(5), 10-14.

Thompson, C., & Sheckley, B.G. (1997). Differences in classroom teaching: Preferences between traditional and adult BSN students. *Journal of Nursing Education, 36*(4), 163-170.

Thompson, J. E. (2002). Competencies for midwifery teachers. *Midwifery, 18*(4), 256-259.

Trevitt, C., Grealish, L., & Reaby, L., (2001). Students in transit: Using a self-directed preceptorship package to smooth the journey. *Journal of Nursing Education, 40*(5), 225.

Trow, M. (1994). Managerialism and the academic profession: The case of England. *Higher Education Policy, 7*(2), 11-18.

Ulloth, J. K. (2003). A qualitative view of humor in nursing classrooms. *Journal of Nursing Education, 42*(3), 125-30.

Usher, K., Nolan, C., Reser, P., Owens, J., & Tollefson, J. (1999). An exploration of the preceptor role: Preceptors' commitment to the preceptor role. *Journal of Advanced Nursing, 29*(2), 506-14.

Viverais-Dresler, G. & Kutschke. (2001). RN student's ratings and opinions related to the importance of certain clinical teacher behaviors. *The Journal of Continuing Education in Nursing, 32*(6), 274-282.

Waring, S. (1996). How part-time, untrained teachers of adults learn to be effective teachers (Doctoral dissertation, Montana State University, 1996). *Dissertation Abstracts International, 57-A,* 2326.

Westra, R.J., & Graziano, M.J. (1992). Preceptors: A comparison of their perceived needs before and after the preceptor experience. *Journal of Continuing Education in Nursing, 23*(5), 212-215.

White, E., Riley, E., Davis, S. & Twinn, S. (1994). *A detailed study of the relationship between teaching, support, supervision and role modeling with the context of Project 2000 courses.* London: English National Board for Nursing, Midwivery and Health Visiting.

Whitehead, D.K. (1997). Characteristics of effective clinical and theory instructors as perceived by LPN to RN versus generic students in an associate degree nursing program (Doctoral dissertation, Florida International University, 1997). *Dissertation Abstracts International.* UMI No. PUZ9726726.

Whitman, N. I. (1990). Clinical colleagues as a source of data for faculty evaluation. *Western Journal of Nursing Research, 12*(5) 644-658.

Wills, M. E. (1997). Link teacher behaviors: Student nurse perceptions. *Nurse Education Today, 17*(3), 232-246.

Wiseman, R. F. (1994). Role model behaviors in the clinical setting. *Journal of Nursing Education, 33*(9), 405-410.

Wong, S. (1978). Nurse-teacher behaviours in the clinical field: Apparent effect on nursing students' learning. *Journal of Advanced Nursing, 3*(4), 369-372.

Young, S., & Shaw, D.G. (1999). Profiles of effective college and university teachers. *The Journal of Higher Education, 70*(6), 670-686.

Yonge, O., Krahn, H., Trojan, L., & Reid, D. (1997). Through the eyes of the preceptor. *Canadian Journal of Nursing Administration, 10*(4), 65-85.

Zimmermann, P. G. (2003). Some practical tips for more effective teaching. *Journal of Emergency Nursing, 29*(3), 283-286.

CHAPTER THREE
FACILITATE LEARNER DEVELOPMENT AND SOCIALIZATION

Effective nurse educators are knowledgeable about learner development and socialization. They understand that each learner has unique needs and ways of being in the world and that there is no single approach to facilitating learner development. Further, nurse educators recognize the value of professional socialization and as a result, create interpersonal relationships and learning environments that assist in the development of a competent professional nurse and an educated citizen.

Based on an understanding of the unique needs of learners for cognitive skills, psychomotor skills, values development, and professional socialization, a variety of assessment techniques and developmental approaches are needed. Nurse educators must possess a solid understanding of the dynamic health care environment, principles of teaching and learning, and the purposes of higher education to effectively socialize students and help them develop to their fullest potential.

To facilitate learner development and socialization effectively the nurse educator:

- Identifies individual learning styles and unique learning needs of international, adult, multicultural, educationally disadvantaged, physically challenged, at-risk, and second degree learners

- Provides resources to diverse learners that help meet their individual learning needs

- Engages in effective advisement and counseling strategies that help learners meet their professional goals

- Creates learning environments that are focused on socialization to the role of the nurse and facilitate learners' self-reflection and personal goal setting

- Fosters the cognitive, psychomotor, and affective development of learners

- Recognizes the influence of teaching styles and interpersonal interactions on learner behaviors and outcomes

- Assists learners to develop the ability to engage in thoughtful and constructive self and peer evaluation

- Models professional behaviors for learners including, but not limited to, involvement in professional organizations, engagement in lifelong learning activities, dissemination of information through publications and presentations, and advocacy

Review of the Literature

Based on results of the literature review conducted for this competency, it is clear that much research is needed in the area of learner development and socialization. There is a particular lack of research in the areas of advisement and counseling, and in how to socialize learners to function in an ever-changing health care environment. There is an extensive amount of anecdotal literature available on these topics. It appears that nurse educators derive a great deal of their knowledge related to the skills and attitudes required to meet learner development and socialization requisites from sharing teaching experiences or reviewing existing literature. Nurse educators have taken the best practices described in the literature and created new approaches to meet learner needs by modifying previously published accounts of teaching experiences. However, research to validate the effectiveness of the many teaching practices related to learner development and socialization is lacking in the literature.

The following discussion represents the five major themes identified from the research literature related to facilitating learner development and socialization. These themes are: assessing learning styles, teaching diverse learners, developing critical thinking skills, socializing learners to the nursing role, and teaching professional values.

Assessing Learning Styles

There is an extensive body of literature in education and psychology related to learning styles. Although nurse educators borrow information related to learning styles from other disciplines and incorporate it into their practice, there is little research to document the utility of this information for nursing education. Since the focus of this book is nursing, the studies presented here represent those that focus on learning styles of nursing students and faculty.

A considerable amount of the literature on learning styles is based on the work of Kolb (1984). To assist the reader in understanding this section on learning styles, Kolb's experiential learning model is briefly described. Kolb's model is based on a belief that all learning occurs in a four-stage cycle. The learner 1) has an immediate or concrete experience, 2) makes an observation and reflects on this experience, 3) assimilates observations and reflections into a theory or concept from which implications for actions are drawn, and 4) tests these implications that serve to create new experiences (Smith & Kolb as cited in Linares, 1999, p. 408).

Based on Kolb's conceptualizations of his experiential learning cycle, he describes four learning style preferences, which stem from learners' inclination to process information either concretely or abstractly or in a reflective or active manner. He names these styles convergers, divergers, assimilators, or accommodators. Very simply, convergers are individuals who prefer abstract conceptualization and active experimentation. Their strength is in complex problem solving, and they would rather focus on the physical rather than the social/personal aspects of a situation. Divergers are learners who rely more on concrete experience and reflective observation. These individuals are creative and imaginative and prefer social and personal aspects of experiences. Assimilators are people who prefer abstract conceptualization and reflective observation. They are strong in inductive reasoning and prefer to focus on ideas and abstraction rather than on people. Finally, accommodators are learners who favor concrete experience with active experimentation. Accommodators are hands-on learners. They are much more intuitive in their response to situations. With this as a basis, the following studies on assessing learning styles are discussed.

Henderson (1996) examined the relationship between learning styles and perceptions of effective teacher characteristics among adult and traditional age learners in a BSN program. Although the study did not demonstrate statistically significant results, the author suggested that it is essential for nurse educators to assess individual learning styles rather than rely solely on preconceived ideas about learners based on their age or other defining characteristics. Also, the author noted that every student group, even those considered traditional learners, is diverse in itself, so educators must be careful not to stereotype or generalize about any group of learners.

Many nurse researchers (Cavanagh, Hogan & Ramgopal, 1995; Haislett, Hughes, Atkinson, & Williams, 1993; Joyce-Nagata, 1996; Laschinger, 1992; Linares, 1999; Rakoczy & Money, 1995) have used Kolb's Learning Style Inventory or derivative instruments to predict the relationship between learners' preferred styles and educational outcomes. The findings of these studies vary specifically depending on the preferred learning style of students. For example in the Haislett et al. study, 74% of the BSN students demonstrated a tendency toward assimilator or diverger styles. However, in the Laschinger study, BSN students tended to consider assimilator and accommodator styles relatively unimportant. In Linares' (1998) study, a preference for the converger style was demonstrated in her sample of generic and RN baccalaureate students. Although logically one can assume that learners are different, the reader might also assume that those who choose nursing as a career have a preferred learning style, given the expectations of the discipline. This assumption, however, has not been demonstrated in the research literature.

Using Kolb's Experiential Learning Theory as a framework, Laschinger (1992) conducted a study to determine the impact of learning environments on adaptive competency development in baccalaureate nursing students. The author determined that nursing learning environments that reflect the importance of people-oriented and scientific skills contributed most to divergent and convergent learning styles. Students in this study considered assimilative styles, such as testing theories, and accommodative styles, such as leading and influencing, to be relatively unimportant to successful functioning in the nursing education environment.

Similar to Laschinger (1992), Cavanagh et al. (1995) used Kolb's Learning Style Inventory to assess student learning styles. The findings of this study reinforced the importance of varying teaching strategies and placing an emphasis on active learning modes such as participation and experiential learning.

Joyce-Nagata (1996) used Kolb's Inventory "to determine the effect of teacher/student learning style congruency on academic performance when controlled for student's previous academic achievement" (p. 69). In this study, traditional-age baccalaureate students, registered nurse baccalaureate students, baccalaureate students holding a previous non-nursing degree, and nursing faculty were compared on learning styles to determine whether faculty and student congruency made a difference in learning outcomes. The results of the study revealed no significant differences in learning styles among the three groups of students. In addition, the learning style differences between faculty and students did not make a difference in the learning outcomes of the students.

Similar to Joyce-Nagata's (1996) study, Linares (1999) focused on understanding whether there was a relationship between learning styles of students and faculty in selected health care professions. Overall, the majority of students preferred the converger style. However, there were some differences by discipline. She found that occupational therapy students were divided equally between convergers and accommodators (37.5%) and between assimilators and divergers (12.5%). Medical technology students were reported to be either convergers or assimilators and physician assistant (PA) students were divided among convergers, assimilators and accommodators. There were no divergers in the PA group.

The purposes of Linares' (1999) study were "to determine if students and faculty in nursing and allied health demonstrate a predominant learning style, if there is a correlation between a specific learning style and self-directedness of these two groups, and if these learning characteristics predict academic success" (p. 409). She found faculty were more self-directed than students, but there was no significant difference between the students and faculty regarding learning style; most were convergers. Learning styles did not predict students' academic success. In contrast to Linares' findings, however, Rakoczy and Money (1995) found that the preferred learning style among nursing students in their study was that of assimilator.

In an effort to determine whether learning style preference affected grade point average, Haislett et al. (1993) conducted a research study with nursing students enrolled in a four-year baccalaureate program. These researchers discovered that assimilator/divergers earned significantly higher grade point averages than accommodators/convergers and, based on the Brown Holtzman Survey of Study Habits, scored higher on the variables of work methods (using the appropriate methods to input and process information) and educational acceptance (students' understandings of the value of the process of higher education and its relevance to their future). Further, the researchers suggest that accommodators are the most at-risk students for academic success for a variety of reasons including, but not limited to, the following: most faculty tend to be abstract learners, accommodators' score lower on the work methods subscale and they prefer to focus on practical application of knowledge and expect results. According to the authors, accommodators want to use information not gather it.

It is easy to see from the studies reported using Kolb's Inventory that the results are inconclusive about the relationship between learning style preferences and learner outcomes.

Future research that includes the replication of studies has the potential to assist nurse educators in understanding the influence of learning style preference on educational outcomes.

In a study completed by Jones, Reichard and Mokhtari (2003), the researchers examined whether preferred learning style is a function of discipline-specific knowledge. In their study, students in English, mathematics, science, and social studies courses completed a version of the Kolb Inventory to discover whether their learning style preference varied based on the discipline. The findings revealed that preferred learning styles are "subject sensitive and that the majority of students perceived different disciplines require different learning strategies, and that they are able to adapt or style-flex to meet the requirements of the learning task" (p. 373). They further discovered that similar to Haislett et al. (1993), assimilators had the highest academic performance. Based on the findings of this study, it is important to examine whether nursing students' learning style preferences change based on the type of learning environment they are in, i.e., clinical vs. theoretical settings, or nursing vs. non-nursing courses.

Andrusyszyn, Cragg, and Humbert (2001) focused on nurse practitioner students' preferences for distance education methods as they relate to learning style, course content, and achievement. A researcher-developed instrument was created to assess students' preferred methods of learning. The authors, in an effort to identify preferred distance learning pedagogy, included items such as the following: 1) I prefer to learn on my own rather than with others; 2) I prefer to learn in smaller groups; 3) I prefer to learn in larger groups; and 4) I prefer to learn by considering the whole picture vs. by focusing on the details. Reliability of the instrument was not established because of the small number of items contained within each preference scale. The researchers reported that there is no single or simple answer to the question of what determines preferences for distance education delivery methods. Students make choices about how they prefer to learn based on a combination of life circumstances, approaches to learning, specific types of content and experiences with technology. Similar to Cavanagh et al. (1995), the authors concluded that delivery methods should be varied when designing distance education courses.

In another study that focused on distance education and learning styles, Carnwell (2000) used grounded theory to understand how different approaches to studying and the need for support and guidance relate to learning via distance technology. The researcher postulated that students use different approaches to interact with learning material based on their preferred learning style. These approaches included systematic wading (reads systematically, avoids shortcuts, may get "bogged down"), speedy focusing (focuses quickly on relevant points, efficient and effective learner), and global dipping (begins systematically but jumps around in the material to find clues, finds learning difficult). The approaches offered give a perspective on how students learn in distance learning situations and should be considered when designing distance education experiences.

The relationship between interface design (usability, visualization, and functionality of web pages) and cognitive style in learning an instructional computer simulation was the focus of a study completed by Effken and Doyle (2001). In this study, the researchers were interested in determining whether cognitive learning style (visual or verbal) affected novices' abilities to use particular computer displays to assimilate information and respond appropriately in specific nursing care simulations. The researchers used three discrete screen displays to illustrate a particular nursing care problem. The displays included: 1) a traditional strip chart of cardiac output, resistance, and arterial and venous pressures plotted as bar graphs, 2) an integrated balloon display showing anatomical constraints on three pressures and cardiac output, and 3) an etiological potentials display integrating three pressures and cardiac output within their potential causes, thus providing a more hierarchical structure of hemodynamic problems available to the clinician. The findings demonstrated that "the effects of cognitive style on performance is mediated by interface design and tended to decrease with practice" (p. 164). Therefore, nurse educators should be cognizant of students' responses to different interface displays and vary them to meet different learner needs.

This review of the research literature on learning styles supports the conclusions Cavanagh and Coffin (1994) drew based on their review of 20 years of research on learning style preference and teaching styles in traditional nursing situations. These researchers concluded that although there is increased motivation in learners whose style matched the teaching methods being used, mixing teaching methods is most desirable as a way to address all learning style preferences.

Teaching Diverse Learners

Even if learning style preferences were the only factor that had to be considered when designing learning experiences, most educators would agree that the challenge of responding to students' needs is complex. In addition to possessing a variety of learning style preferences, nursing students bring a great deal of individual diversity to both classroom and clinical settings. For the purpose of this review, diversity includes learners who are international, multicultural, adult, nontraditional, educationally disadvantaged, at-risk, physically challenged, or seeking a second degree. This list is not exhaustive, nor is each of the categories distinct. The intent here is to help the reader understand the complex nature of learners and identify the unique skills and attitudes that are needed to meet the teaching challenges such diversity creates.

Students with disabilities present unique needs in the learning environment. Carroll (2004) stated that nursing education has a legal and ethical obligation to provide an education to qualified students who have physical disabilities. However, the students' experiences may not be positive when they seek admission to nursing programs. Maheady (1999) conducted a qualitative study to describe the experiences of nursing students with disabilities (visual, auditory, or physical impairment). The study focused on admission and accommodation guidelines and disabled students' experiences with faculty, patients, nurses, and other students. The results of the study demonstrated that admission guidelines are often not upheld despite the fact that nurse educators have the responsibility of upholding federal laws ensuring that students have equal access to the nursing profession [and] to make admission and retention decisions that promote successful student outcomes as well as patient safety" (p. 169).

This study also demonstrated that accommodation documents existed in all nursing programs included in the study. Students corroborated that the accommodations included in the documents were provided. However, they also shared that, at times, these accommodations had a negative impact on classmates. Disabled students reported the need to cope with negative attitudes that remain pervasive in society. They verbalized that faculty, peers, patients, and nurses continue to present pessimistic and negative views of disability. Students reported that disclosure of their disability frequently resulted in negative outcomes and that it was their desire to be treated based on their abilities (Maheady, 1999).

Extensive research has been conducted in education on the unique needs of the learning disabled. A study completed by Graves, Landers, Lokerson, Luchow and Horvath (1993) provided a list of competencies designed to prepare teachers to educate students with learning disabilities. This study used a two-round Delphi technique to create the list of competencies. The list is divided into 10 discrete areas. Each section describes the knowledge and skill competencies needed by the educator to work with learning disabled students regardless of discipline. The 10 major areas include: nature and needs of students with learning disabilities; academic support areas such as study skills, consumer skills, and career/vocational skills; curriculum for support areas and modifications of school core curriculum; assessment, methods, use, and interpretation; classroom assessment, management, and motivation; collaborative and consulting skills; specialized instructional strategies, technologies, and materials; historical and legal aspects; nontraditional practices and procedures; and clinical/ field experiences. The competencies included in the list provide some important considerations for nurse educators.

Kolanko (2003) used a qualitative approach to describe the meaning of being a nursing student with a learning disability. In this study, the researcher used case studies to understand the unique experiences of students with learning disabilities and found that these experiences centered around five themes: 1) struggling; 2) learning how to learn with a learning disability; 3) managing time; 4) receiving social support, and 5) telling personal stories. The participants all had average to above average intellectual functioning. Learning disabled students noted that "direct instruction, structure, consistency, clear directions, organization, and a positive instructor attitude assisted their learning." (p. 251). Most educators would agree that these same concepts are important to all students, not only those with a learning disability.

Culturally diverse students may also present with unique learning needs. Several research studies were found that addressed the needs of culturally diverse students. Saenz, Wyatt, and Reinard (1998), speech and language pathologists, made the case that university faculty need to be increasingly aware of the needs and expectations of minority students. To help educators understand their role with minority students, the authors conducted a study designed to assess students' perceptions of factors related to academic success. The results indicated that students perceived their academic success could be improved by directing more attention toward financial support, mentoring, faculty development especially as it relates to learning expectation discrepancies and communication styles, cooperative learning, and other interactive, student-centered strategies.

In a study by Yoder (1996), nurse educators (N = 26) were interviewed regarding the approaches they use when teaching ethnically diverse students. The author also interviewed ethnic graduate nurses (N = 17) from populations that are under-represented in nursing programs. The findings from this grounded theory study revealed the positive and negative consequences of the patterns of interaction between nurse educators and students from varying cultural backgrounds. The labels given to the patterns of response included: generic (response based on a low level of cultural awareness), mainstreaming (response is based on a belief that students' problems are a result of their lack of understanding of the majority culture), culturally nontolerant (response indicates unwillingness to tolerate cultural differences and exhibits behaviors that create barriers), struggling (response demonstrates an increasing level of cultural awareness with attendant struggle to modify teaching/learning environment in order to support culturally diverse students), and bridging (response indicates high level of cultural awareness and adaptation of teaching/learning methods to respond to students' needs). The majority of the students indicated that they did not experience the bridging pattern in their interactions with faculty; the majority of the students also indicated that they had experienced the culturally nontolerant pattern in their interactions with faculty. An understanding of the response patterns can assist nurse educators in creating a positive learning environment for culturally diverse students. It also emerged that students' perceptions may be influenced by the degree of barriers or the level of need they are experiencing (e.g., financial, language, academic, cultural). Students cited having ethnically diverse faculty as role models to be an important need in nursing education.

Several authors have looked at specific multicultural populations. Yurovich (2001), for example, conducted a grounded theory study that focused on identifying the barriers American Indian students experience in attempting to complete programs of study. Through constant comparative analysis of 18 interviews, Yurovich found four interactive core variables (the individual American Indian student, the instructor, the institutional environment, and external influences) and seven properties that support academic success (focus on goals, adjust to dominant culture, invest in self-assessment, develop assertiveness skills, establish a support community, socialize into roles of student and nurse, and master the content) that emerged. Yurovich stated that the variables and properties create a gestalt that facilitates students' academic success. The author concluded that if faculty develop learning situations that attend to the core variables and support the seven properties, student success is more likely.

Nahas (2000) studied the unique needs of Jordanian students in the learning environment. This study was part of a larger research project that "discovered, described, explained, and compared Australian and Jordanian nursing students' caring and non-caring encounters with their clinical teachers" (p. 257). According to Nahas, "findings revealed that Jordanian nursing students reported their clinical experiences as beneficial when their encounters with clinical teachers were conducted through mothering, translating, sustaining, negotiating and transforming processes" (p. 257). Participants described mothering behaviors as "guiding, protecting, assisting, understanding and supporting" (p. 262). Translating and sustaining were equated to the mothering theme. Faculty were seen as individuals who nourished students and helped them learn in the clinical environment. Negotiating was described as the way faculty paved the way for students to "blend in" in the clinical area. Transforming reflected a metamorphosis for students in which the faculty-student relationship assisted them in learning that only through self-determination and feelings of self-worth would they value their career choice. This is particularly important given the low status of nursing in Jordan.

Canales and Bowers (2001) used grounded theory to study Latina nurse educators' perceptions about cultural competence. The study's purpose was to define what cultural competence means from the perspective of Latina nurse educators, and how these perceptions impact their teaching practices with students. The researchers interviewed 10 doctorally prepared Latina nurse educators. The results of this study revealed that Latina nurse educators did not differentiate between culturally competent care and competence. Rather, they considered competence to include cultural competence, and that "differences" among individuals may not solely be defined as "cultural" differences. These educators stated they use teaching strategies that teach students to respect all individuals who may be perceived to be "different;" a frequently used strategy was to create a context by which student perceptions about "differences" may be changed. Community learning experiences were commonly used to create this context. A cited limitation of the study is that it did not include student perceptions about the effectiveness of the teaching practices used by the Latina nurse educators.

In a study that addressed the unique needs of international students, Carty, O'Grady, Wichaikhum and Bull (2002) found that international nursing students pursuing doctoral degrees lacked familiarity with the U.S. health care system and had limited experience with seminars as a teaching/learning strategy. These students also reported limited opportunities to participate in faculty research and that they struggled with expected course loads. The findings suggested that nurse educators may need to help international students learn very basic things (e.g., what a seminar is) before they address course material.

Based on a review of 18 years of literature on international graduate nursing students, Julian, Keane and Davidson (1999) concluded that students require writing support, second-language acquisition skills, phonology, discourse analysis, and language pragmatics to identify unique social and language phenomena. Nurse educators are best prepared to teach international students if they recognize the students' fundamental needs to communicate effectively and to engage in social relationships, as well as cope with cultural differences, while they pursue graduate education in nursing in the United States.

Moffitt and Wuest (2002) made the case that "most of the research and theoretical literature to date has focused on identifying the beliefs, values and traditions of specific cultures and on developing assessment tools" (p. 108) with the specific purpose of helping students provide culturally sensitive care. The researchers suggested there is a need for educators to develop multicultural classrooms where students develop "culturally responsive behaviors that validate cultural identity and enhance cultural caring both in the classroom and clinical areas" (p. 107). To address their concerns, the researchers used an evaluation model to assess the cultural component of one nursing program's curriculum. Findings revealed that it is important to include traditional knowledge of individual differences in "multicultural classrooms and practice settings through open dialogue, sharing circles, cultural conflict resolution, and the development of relationships based on the integration of the cultural model" (p. 115).

Although St. Clair and McKenry's (1999) research does not focus on how to teach multicultural students, their study of senior nursing students did address how to overcome ethnocentrism. These researchers asserted that cultural immersion experiences help students develop cultural competence and reduce cultural ethnocentrism, and therefore should be provided for all students.

The research literature on diverse learners demonstrates the many ways in which learners are different, and illustrates the complex set of skills that are required of nurse educators to meet the needs of these diverse learners. The literature also provides the opportunity for nurse educators to explore the varying definitions and descriptions of diversity and identify teaching/learning strategies that will be most effective in meeting these students' learning needs.

Developing Learners' Critical Thinking Skills

As part of developing and socializing the learner, nurse educators must have a well-honed ability to assist nursing students in the development of critical thinking skills. Critical thinking skills have been demonstrated to be essential in the development of high quality nursing professionals. As a concept, it is of significant interest to nurse educators. The value of critical thinking and its relationship to practice has been studied extensively within nursing and other disciplines. Simpson and Courtney (2002) completed an extensive review of the literature on critical thinking in nursing. They offered definitions, components, and dimensions of critical thinking. They further explored the literature on the similarities and differences between critical thinking, problem-solving, decision-making, and creative thinking. Finally, they offered a list of strategies for teaching critical thinking that included works by Elliott (1996), Abegglen (1997), Morin (1997), Oermann (1997), Whiteside (1997), Lipmann and Deatrick (1997), Lenberg (1997), Daly (1998), Schell (1998), Sellappah, Hussey, Blackmore, and McMurray (1998), Fowler (1998) and Billings and Halstead (1998). For this review, the research literature has been examined to determine ways in which nurse educators can create learning situations that facilitate students' critical thinking.

There is a great deal of consistency in the literature that supports the idea that the development of critical thinking skills is a process. Duchscher (2003) interviewed five newly graduated baccalaureate nurses to "explore how [they] perceived critical thinking" (p. 16) and how undergraduate education can facilitate critical thinking in relation to the practice of nursing. The author concluded that the following strategies encourage critical thinking: 1) teaching students the elements, principles, and characteristics of critical thinkers; 2) consistently demonstrating the elements, principles, and characteristics of critical thinking; 3) encouraging a critical approach to thinking in class and clinical, and 4) fostering an environment where challenging the teacher is accepted. Teaching students to question existing theories and ideas assists in the deconstruction and reconstruction of the kind of knowledge that leads to new discoveries.

In a pilot study, Bell et al. (2002) similarly used qualitative methodology to evaluate the effectiveness of a six-step critical thinking process described by Thornhill and Wafer (1997). In the first step, students describe a critical incident in clinical that caused them to engage in critical thinking. In step two, students respond to four questions related to the critical incident: What triggered the critical thinking? What resources were helpful? What were the high and low points? What happened as a result of your critical thinking? In step three, students identify explicit and implicit assumptions in the incident. Step four requires the students to examine the contextual variables and how different perspectives influence their thinking. Step five asks the students to speculate on alternative ways that the incident might have happened. Finally, in step six, students are asked to identify clinical practice issues found in the incident and assess the influence of the critical thinking strategy on their learning. The authors concluded that "the six step learning strategy delineates a process of critical thinking applicable to nursing" (p. 77) and it helped students examine their assumptions and include context in the analysis of clinical situations. Since examining assumptions is characteristic of critical thinking, this six-step process would seem to have some value in promoting critical thinking.

Kuiper (2002) examined the use of self-regulated learning strategies to enhance metacognition. "Self-regulated learning (SRL) is a synthesis of the academic research supporting the conceptual relationships of metacognitive and behavioral processes, and environmental structuring for educational settings" (p. 80). She used a comparative descriptive design to "describe the effects of SRL prompts on the cognitive processes of baccalaureate-degree and associate-degree nurses in clinical settings with the pedagogical strategy of reflective journaling" (p. 80). Novice BSN-prepared nurses (N = 18) and novice ADN-prepared nurses (N = 14) wrote journal entries for eight weeks as part of preceptorship programs in five different acute care clinical settings. These journals were analyzed using a verbal protocol analysis as the framework for decoding cognitive processes. Intercoder reliability for this study was reported as 80%. As a result of the analysis, Kuiper offered the opinion that critical thinking skills are integrated within self-regulation strategies and that prompting self-regulation can increase students' critical thinking. Reflective journaling is one example of a teaching strategy that enhances metacognition.

In a similar study, Martin (2002) included students from BSN and ADN nursing programs to test a mid-range theory of critical thinking of nurses. Martin was interested in examining the level of critical thinking used and the quality of decisions made by BSN students, ADN students, nonlicensed graduates, and expert nurses. In this descriptive, correlational study, she collected data on 149 individuals and found that as clinical experience increased, so did the individual's ability to critically think as measured by the Elements of Thought Instrument (ETI). Validity and reliability (Cronbach's alpha of 0.96) were established for the ETI. These findings were supported based on her comparisons of nursing students to clinical experts. Specifically, Martin states that "as nurses achieve higher levels of clinical expertise, they use more critical thinking during a decision-making situation as predicted by the Theory of Critical Thinking of Nurses. Factors such as knowledge and experience, thought to influence the level of clinical expertise, may contribute to increased critical thinking" (p. 246). This finding supports the work of other authors who have reported that familiarity with the situation enhances critical thinking.

Some researchers have focused their study of critical thinking on practicing nurses to identify the educational value of promoting critical thinking in students. Profetto-McGrath, Hesketh, Lang, and Estabrooks (2003) were interested in the relationship between critical thinking and research utilization among practicing nurses (N = 141) and found a statistically significant positive correlation between research utilization and critical thinking disposition as measured by Facione and Facione's (1992) California Critical Thinking Dispositions Inventory (CCTDI). They determined that "nurses who have the attributes consistent with the ideal critical thinker…are more likely to use research findings in their work as nurses" (p. 334). The researchers stated that "these findings indicate a need to foster critical thinking in both nursing education and the work environment" (p. 322).

Tsui (2002) used case study analysis to examine educational practices that facilitate critical thinking, specifically the relationship between pedagogy and the development of critical thinking. She asserted that one cannot remove the concept from the environment. To support her position, the researcher made site visits to four higher education institutions to conduct a comparative analysis of instructional differences found at the institutions. She primarily collected the data through interviews of administrators, faculty and students, and classroom observations. For the purpose of the study, critical thinking was defined as "students abilities' to identify issues and assumptions, recognize important relationships, make correct inferences, evaluate evidence or authority, and deduce conclusions" (p. 743). Tsui's analysis of the qualitative data indicated that the development of critical thinking is linked to an emphasis on writing and rewriting at the analysis and synthesis levels. She also determined that using discussion as a teaching method helps build critical thinking abilities. Tsui asserted that "widespread efforts to heighten students' critical thinking through instructional change are more likely to come about if they involve altering commonplace teaching techniques rather than radically replacing them" (p. 754). Tsui identified some study limitations to be the potential influence of an outside observer in the classroom on student and faculty behaviors, the lack of an objective means to measure students' critical thinking, and the fact that the definition of critical thinking used for the study was somewhat narrow in scope and did not include problem-solving.

Duchscher (2003) conducted a qualitative study to explore how female, newly graduated baccalaureate nurses perceived critical thinking. In this study, the researcher conducted in-depth interviews with five newly graduated nurses between the ages of 22 and 25. She also asked the new graduates to engage in writing a reflective journal on a monthly basis. Evidence suggested that the participants did not necessarily connect critical thinking to having a spirit of inquiry, but rather had a more prescriptive, reductionistic approach to their practice. Duchscher stated that the study provides insights into the role of undergraduate education in teaching and fostering critical thinking as an approach to nursing practice. All participants were educated in a "behaviorist" paradigm of learning where behavior change was the primary indicator learning had occurred. Traditionally, this way of thinking promotes an orientation toward task performance, rather than towards cognitively driven questioning of theoretical constructs that support the desired behavior (p. 24). Duchscher concluded by challenging nurse educators to teach critical thinking, but also to model an attitude of inquiry that creates an environment where discovery is an accepted practice rather than one that is unusual.

Chau et al. (2001) examined the use of videotaped vignettes as a teaching method to enhance critical thinking in clinical situations. Despite insignificant findings from this pre-test/post-test study, the authors concluded that students found the use of vignettes to be a highly desirable learning strategy for preparing them for the clinical setting. In a similar approach, Neill,, Lachat and Taylor-Panek (1997) used case studies to enhance critical thinking skills. Faculty added group exploration of patient case studies to a lecture in a sophomore nursing process course. While no specific data were provided to support the assertion, the authors stated that they believed the group format facilitated higher-level analysis of the case studies and improved utilization of the nursing process. The faculty enjoyed the teaching strategy and the majority of the students (70%) had positive comments about the group case study work.

Myrick and Yonge (2001) conducted a grounded theory study to identify the key elements of a climate that supports critical thinking, describe important insights into the roles of the preceptor and staff within that context, and discuss how nursing faculty can more actively contribute to ensuring that the learning climate supports development of critical thinking skills. The authors reported that when preceptors genuinely value, support, and work with students in the practice setting and the staff accept preceptors as part of the team, a climate conducive to learning and critical thinking is established. Myrick and Yonge contended that the impact of the learning environment on students' abilities to critically think during preceptorship experiences must be valued.

In a more recent study by Myrick and Yonge (2004), the researchers examined the process used in the preceptorship experience to enhance critical thinking at the graduate level. The result was the development of a grounded theory named the Relational Process, which indicates that specific preceptor behaviors are essential to enhance critical thinking of graduate nursing students. These behaviors include respect, flexibility, openness, safety/trust, and skepticism.

Sellappah, Hussey, Blackmore, and McMurray (1998) examined questioning as a strategy for developing critical thinking. Findings of this work revealed that critical thinking is increased when educators ask questions that require analysis, synthesis, and evaluation. The authors suggested that the clinical area is an ideal place to develop critical thinking skills using questioning techniques.

The literature on critical thinking is extensive. Despite the volumes of research conducted on the concept, there is limited understanding of critical thinking and its implementation in nursing. In addition, there has been little attention to building on the research literature that already exists. For nurse educators to effectively facilitate critical thinking some common understanding of what is known is important. According to Tanner (2005) the literature has demonstrated:

- critical thinking and clinical thinking are different constructs and the evidence does not support a relationship between theses skills,

- our measurement of critical thinking has not kept pace with our conceptualizations of it, and

- we have not been able to demonstrate a significant improvement in critical thinking as a result of instruction (p. 48).

The review conducted for this chapter contributes some additional insights, including that the environment mostly likely to facilitate development of critical thinking is one in which the learner is provided with the opportunity to be self-directed, encouraged to question assumptions and prevailing understanding without fear of judgment, and supported through teaching strategies that facilitate higher-order thinking.

Based on these conclusions, nursing education researchers will be challenged to further develop the environments in which critical thinking is most likely to be enhanced and demonstrate that indeed it does make a difference.

Socializing Learners to the Nursing Role

It is our responsibility as educators to create environments in which learning can occur. However, there is little published research that documents how such an environment can be created. In addition, there is even less research literature on how to socialize students to the nursing role. Similar to the majority of research published about learning styles, the limited amount of knowledge about creating effective learning environments appears to be derived from modifying personal experiences reported by others, rather than being derived from research. This section summarizes the research that was found related to creating environments for learning and socializing the learner into the nursing role.

Although a number of studies imply that creation of a learning environment is important, only one study was found that specifically addressed this area. In a mixed method study, Schaefer and Zygmont (2003) examined teaching styles of 187 nurse educators to determine whether they were teacher-centered or student-centered. Subjects completed a Principles of Adult Learning instrument to measure their teaching style. Previously, reliability and validity of the instrument have been established. Reliability of the instrument for this study was .78. Schaefer and Zygmont's quantitative analyses revealed that faculty in this study were more teacher-centered. However, analysis of the narrative data, which consisted of written philosophies of teaching and learning by the study participants, revealed that faculty held more student-centered beliefs about teaching and learning than the quantitative data indicated. Recommendations from the study included supporting new faculty as they make the transition from clinician to teacher, developing mentoring relationships for new faculty, creating opportunities for faculty to discuss barriers that impede student-centered teaching, and eliminating these barriers.

In a phenomenological study by Beck (1993), students' perceptions of their first clinical experience were examined. The findings of this study demonstrated the importance of creating an environment for learning. Specifically, Beck addressed the importance of creating a learning environment, one where the emphasis is on learning and not on perfection. Beck reiterated the conclusions from Burnard's (1992) study that described the value of reflection in helping students assimilate into the clinical practice arena. Further, Burnhard and Beck agree that role modeling in the clinical site is essential to assist students with their transition from students to clinicians.

Wong, Kam, and Lee (2000) conducted a study similar to Beck's (1993). In this study, the researchers were interested in understanding the lived experiences of beginning nursing students in Hong Kong. Phenomenological analysis was used to understand the process of professional socialization. The findings highlighted the importance of providing a clinical learning environment that is conducive to learning and supports positive personal relationships and professional development. The researchers conclude that a positive learning experience affirms one's career choice, whereas a negative experience diminishes the student's career choice and leads to feelings of dissatisfaction ultimately leading to departure from the profession.

Beck (1991) conducted a study to identify students' perceptions of caring faculty. The themes that emerged from this phenomenological analysis included: attentive presence (focusing on the student), sharing of selves (giving time, sharing emotions, acting nonjudgmentally), and consequences (making the student feel respected and valued, demonstrating caring interactions, reminiscing). Dillon and Stines (1996) also studied students' perceptions of caring. In this study, the authors stated that caring is taught primarily through modeling behaviors. The results of these studies provide valuable insights into the importance of creating and reinforcing caring student-faculty interactions as one means of socializing students into the nursing profession.

Professional socialization of students is important, as discussed in many journal articles and nursing texts. However, the literature lacks a consistent definition of socialization and best practices for facilitating socialization to the nursing profession, thus leading to difficulty in developing ideal socialization experiences for students. The research articles found in the literature provide a glimpse of the work that has been conducted as well as ideas for future directions.

Cook, Gilmer, and Bess (2003) believed that students have a framework for professional identity before they begin nursing courses, so they used a qualitative design to examine beginning students' definitions of nursing. The authors stated, "nursing identity is a developmental process that evolves throughout professional nurses' careers" (p. 311). In the study, they found that students described nursing in different ways. One way is as a verb: caring, nurturing, teaching, implementing, assessing/analyzing, advocating, and managing. Another is as a noun: profession, holistic system, connecting system, delivery system, and as a discipline. A third way is as a transaction: health promotion, treatment of illness, prevention of illness, and promotion of self-care. The researchers postulated that if nurse educators know and understand students' perceptions, they can build experiences into the curriculum that expand and support the ideas students hold.

Socialization in nursing can mean different things to different individuals. It is particularly difficult to identify a consistent definition or process for the socialization of nursing students. In addition, how a program is planned and implemented may impact the socialization process. Eckhardt (2002) examined "the effects of program design on the bureaucratic and professional role conceptions of registered nurses in baccalaureate nursing programs" (p. 157). Recent graduates from three different baccalaureate nursing programs were included in the study.

Specifically, the research question for the study was: "Are there differences in the role conceptions of graduating RN students who experience different processes of organizational socialization in generic, RN-track and second-step baccalaureate nursing programs?" (p. 159). The theory of organizational socialization developed by Van Maanen and Schein (1979) for use in educational contexts was the framework for the study. This model describes six processes that interact to influence learning and the development of either professional or bureaucratic behaviors: collective vs. individual emphasis; formal vs. informal emphasis; sequential vs. random steps; fixed vs. variable timetables; serial vs. disjunctive emphasis, and investiture vs. divestiture emphasis. Findings indicated that there were significant differences ($p < .05$) in role conceptions depending upon the program from which the students graduated. According to Eckhardt, attending to the processes (individual, informal, random, disjunctive, and investiture processes) that promote role innovation and a high level of professional development can assist program planning for professional socialization of students. Specifically, she suggested some educational practice implications including: tailoring program requirements to individuals, relating classroom learning to professional practice experience, allowing flexibility in learning experiences, exposing RNs to diverse ideas, and confirming their previous learning and professional experience.

In a qualitative research study on professional role transition for graduate nurses, Thomka (2001) presented a case for mentoring as an appropriate strategy for moving graduate nurses into the role of a professional. Sixteen registered nurses completed a questionnaire about their experiences during their first year of practice post-graduation. They were asked to provide information about how they felt they were treated by their peers, including examples of how they were treated in ways that were helpful and in ways that were not helpful. They also provided suggestions for an "ideal" transition. Seven of the sixteen nurses suggested a mentor would be helpful during the transition period. Although the researcher did not address the use of mentoring as a socialization technique for nursing students, it may be a strategy that can lead to positive outcomes in the socialization of students as well.

Crawford, Dresen, and Tschikota (2000) studied the role of the preceptor in facilitating learning and socialization. They conducted a phenomenological study and found that students believed that developing a productive relationship, creating a safe environment for learning, teaching strategies employed by the preceptor, and soloing all helped their learning. The researchers reported that understanding students' experiences with preceptors will help the nurse educator to create a supportive learning environment.

More research on socialization and role development in nursing education is needed, as the studies currently reported in the literature are limited. It is essential that programs of research be developed to further the understanding of how nurse educators can create learning experiences to fully develop the student for the role of professional nurse.

Teaching Professional Values

Nursing education programs often include in their philosophies or organizational statements declarations about values. These program philosophies usually include statements that address the need to provide values-based care, facilitate students' learning professional nursing values, or respect the values of students in the educational process. Despite the inclusion of values-related statements in such documents, there has been little attention to defining what educators are referring to when they address the term "values" or how nurse educators are prepared to engage their students in activities that support the acquisition of values. This section explores the limited research available on how nurse educators teach students specifically about values, which is an important component of professional socialization.

In response to the acknowledged paucity of literature on the development of professional nursing values, Eddy, Elfrink, Weise, and Schank (1994) conducted a study to determine if there were different perceptions about professional nursing values between senior baccalaureate nursing students and their faculty. The Professional Nursing Behavior Instrument (PNB), a researcher-developed instrument based on the nursing role behaviors identified in the AACN's (1986) Essentials Report, was used. Reliability of the instrument was previously established with a Cronbach's alpha of .89 for the total instrument. Role subscale alphas for this study ranged from .66 to .83. The findings revealed that faculty values were significantly higher (p <.045) than students' values. This should not be a surprise, given that faculty are socialized to the role of the nurse. The authors also discovered that enrollment in courses in ethics, theology, and philosophy did not significantly affect student values.

According to Mayo (1996), nurse educators are responsible for preparing future nurses for community-based practice by instilling moral and professional practice obligations, cultural sensitivity, and other facets of social responsibility. She conducted a qualitative research study to illustrate the concept of social responsibility and how it is developed during a clinical practicum in a large urban homeless shelter. Undergraduate nursing students (N = 33) maintained a journal reflecting upon their experiences in the homeless shelter. The students' narratives provided important insight into what students think about concepts such as social responsibility. Specifically, Mayo supported extended contact with at-risk populations in the community, as she believes that students are better able to analyze and critique health care issues and recommend social change when they work with at-risk populations in the community, thus developing professional values. She also recommended journaling as an effective teaching strategy for addressing the affective domain of learning.

Thorpe and Loo's (2003) study of 152 undergraduate nursing students' values profiles as compared to 111 undergraduate management students' values profiles revealed that the nursing students "fit the occupational stereotype and sex-type norms associated with nursing, recognizing the high value placed on altruism and professionalism" (p. 88). The students' values profiles were determined by the 100-item Life Roles Inventory-Values Scale. Alpha coefficients for the values scales ranged from .63 to .90. Nursing students indicated that the values of personal development and altruism were most important to them and the values of cultural identity, risk, creativity, and physical prowess were least important. The authors proposed that nurse educators should provide students with opportunities to self-assess personal values early in their educational experiences so that they can ascertain if they want to actively work to change their values. Nurse educators may also wish to design learning experiences that assist in value development, for example, teaching risk management skills and fostering creativity.

Many nurse educators would agree with Glenn's (1999) statement that, "effective interpersonal collaboration depends upon establishing understanding that respects differences in values and beliefs, and thus differences in response to the multiplicity of patient/client/user needs" (p. 202). Despite this recognized need, little attention has been given to these differences in professional education. Research needs to be conducted regarding the development and integration of teaching/learning strategies that support an understanding of and respect for personal and professional values.

Identified Gaps in the Literature

The research related to the knowledge, skills, and attitudes required of nursing educators to facilitate learner development and socialization has been limited. It is clear that additional research is needed to fully understand the complexity of learning styles, strategies useful to facilitate diverse learner needs, and the most effective ways to provide advisement and counseling to nursing students. Another important question that needs to be addressed through research is the extent to which theories borrowed from other disciplines have relevance for nursing education. As the discipline seeks highly qualified individuals to assume roles as nurse educators, research must be completed that will help them develop the competencies necessary to provide excellent learning experiences for students. To that end, research that focuses on the varying aspects of the nurse educator role will be essential.

More research needs to be focused on how nurse educators can facilitate learners' abilities to practice effectively in an ever-changing health care environment. Specifically, what are the essential skills that students will need to remain agile in rapidly changing systems, and what are the best ways to help students develop those skills?

It will also be important to conduct more research on the dynamic of the teaching/learning environment. Nurse educators need to understand how teaching styles, learning environments, and interpersonal interactions promote or impede successful learning outcomes. With regard to our understanding of values development in the professional nurse, nursing education scholars need to explore the strategies that enhance values development and how best to measure student progress in this area.

Research will also be needed in the area of diversity. These studies will need to address the multiplicity of diversities suggested in this review. Educators may need to first develop conceptual clarity on the many types of diversity they face in the classroom and in the clinical area.

Finally, successful facilitation of learning requires educators to have knowledge of the legal and ethical issues regarding students and the educational environment. Considering the potential complexity of legal and ethical issues related to student performance in a practice discipline, it is surprising that these topics are not addressed with more frequency in the literature.

Priorities for Future Research

In nursing education classrooms across the country and in many places in the world, nursing students are being taught the value of evidenced-based clinical practice. How can nurse educators teach their students the importance of evidenced-based practice if their own teaching practices are not evidence-based? It is essential that nurse educators continue to conduct pedagogical research and implement the findings of such studies if they are to be most effective in facilitating learner development and socialization.

- What skills are needed by educators to effectively accommodate individual learning style preferences of students in the classroom and clinical settings?
- What are the most effective advising and counseling strategies that faculty can use to assist students?
- What are the most successful strategies to facilitate the learning needs of diverse learners?
- What are the most effective ways to facilitate the professional socialization of students?
- What are the most effective ways to facilitate values development in nursing students?
- What are the relationships among teaching style, learning style, and learning outcomes?
- What is critical thinking in nursing and how do educators facilitate its development in nursing students?
- What are nurse educators' understanding of the legal and ethical issues related to students and the educational environment?

References

Abegglen, J. (1997). Critical thinking in nursing: Classroom tactics that work. *Journal of Nursing Education,* 36(10), 452-458.

American Association of Colleges of Nursing. (1986). *The essentials of baccalaureate education for professional nursing practice.* Washington, DC: Author.

Andrusyszyn, M,, Cragg, B. E. & Humert, J. (2001). Nurse practitioner preferences for distance education methods related to learning styles, course content, and achievement. *Journal of Nursing Education, 40*(4), 163-170.

Bartlett, D. J., & Cox, P. D. (2002). Measuring change in students' critical thinking ability: Implications for health care education. *Journal of Allied Health,* 31(2), 64-69.

Beck, C. T. (1991). How students perceive faculty caring: A phenomenological study. *Nurse Educator, 16*(5), 18-22.

Beck, C. T. (1993). Nursing students' initial clinical experience: A phenomenological study. *International Journal of Nursing Studies, 30*(6), 489-497.

Bell, M. L., Heye, M. L., Campion, L, Hendricks, P. B., Owens, B. L., Schoonover, J. (2002). Evaluation of a process-focused learning strategy to promote critical thinking. *Journal of Nursing Education, 41*(4), 175-177.

Billings, D. M. & Halstead, J. A. (1998). *Teaching in nursing: A faculty guide.* Philadelphia: Saunders.

Burnard, P. (1992). Learning from experience: Nurse tutors' and student nurses' perceptions of experiential learning in nursing education: Some initial findings. *International Journal of Nursing Studies, 29*(2), 151-161.

Canales, M. K, & Bowers, B. J. (2001). Expanding conceptualizations of cultural competent care. *Journal of Advanced Nursing, 36*(1), 102-111.

Carnwell, R. (2000). Approaches to study and their impact on the need for support and guidance in distance learning. *Open Learning, 15*(2), 123-140.

Carroll, S. (2004). Inclusion of people with physical disabilities in nursing education. *Journal of Nursing Education, 43*(5), 207-212.

Carty, R., O'Grady, E.T., Wichaikhum, O, & Bull, J. (2002). Opportunities in preparing global leaders in nursing. *Journal of Professional Nursing, 18*(2), 70-77.

Cavanagh, S. J., & Coffin, D.A. (1994). Matching instructional preference and teaching style: Review of the literature. *Nurse Education Today, 14*(2), 106-110.

Cavanagh, S. J., Hogan, K. & Ramgopal, T. (1995). The assessment of student nurse learning styles using the Kolb learning style inventory. *Nurse Education Today, 15*(3), 177-183.

Chau, J. P. C., Chang, A. M., Lee, I. F. K., Ip, W.Y., Lee, D. T. F., & Wootton, Y. (2001). Effects of using videotaped vignettes on enhancing students' critical thinking ability in a baccalaureate nursing programme. *Journal of Advanced Nursing, 36*(1), 112-119.

Cook, T. H., Gilmer, M. J., & Bess, C. J. (2003). Beginning students' definitions of nursing: An inductive framework of professional identity. *Journal of Nursing Education, 42*(7), 311-317.

Crawford, M. J., Dresen, S. E., & Tsckikota, S.E. (2000). From 'getting to know you' to 'soloing': The preceptor-student relationship. *NT Research, 5*(1), 5-20.

Daly, W. M. (1998). Critical thinking as an outcome of nursing education. Why is it important to nursing practice? *Journal of Advanced Nursing, 28*(2), 323-331.

Dillion, R. S., & Stines, P.W. (1996). A phenomenological study of faculty-student caring interactions. *Journal of Nursing Education, 35*(3), 113-118.

Duchscher, J.E. B. (2003). Critical thinking: Perceptions of newly graduated female baccalaureate nurses. *Journal of Nursing Education, 42*(1), 14-26.

Eckhardt, J.A. (2002). Effects of program design on the professional socialization of RN-BSN students. *Journal of Professional Nursing, 18*(3), 157-164.

Eddy, D.M., Elfrink, V., Weise, D., & Schank, M. J. (1994). Importance of professional nursing values: A national study of baccalaureate programs. *Journal of Nursing Education, 33(6), 257-262.*

Effken, J. & Doyle, M. (2001). Interface design and cognitive style in learning an instructional computer simulation. *Computers in Nursing, 19*(4), 164-171.

Elliott, D. (1996). Promoting critical thinking in the classroom. *Nurse Educator, 21*(2), 49-52.

Facione, P. A. & Facione, N. C. (1992). *The California Critical Thinking Disposition Inventory.* Millbrae, CA: California Academic Press.

Fowler, L. P. (1998). Improving critical thinking in nursing practice. *Journal of Staff Development,14*(4), 183-187.

Glenn, S. (1999). Educating for interprofessional collaboration: Teaching about values. *Nursing Ethics, 6*(3), 202-213.

Graves, A., Landers, M. F., Lokerson, J., Luchow, J., & Horvath, M. (1993). The development of a competency list for teachers of students with learning disabilities. *Learning Disabilities Research and Practice, 8*(3), 188-199.

Haislett, J., Hughes, R. B., Atkinson, G., & Williams, C. L. (1993). Success in baccalaureate nursing programs: A matter of accommodation? *Journal of Nursing Education, 32*(2), 64-70.

Henderson, I. T.(1996). Learning styles and perceptions of effective teacher characteristics among adult and traditional learners in baccalaureate nursing programs. (UMI No. PPUZ97098)

Jones, C., Reichard, C., & Mokhtari, K. (2003). Are students' learning styles discipline specific? *Community College Journal of Research and Practice, 27*(5), 363-376.

Joyce-Nagata, B. (1996). Students' academic performance in nursing as a function of student and faculty learning style congruency. *Journal of Nursing Education, 35*(2), 69-73.

Julian, M. A., Keane, A. & Davidson, K. (1999). Language Plus for international graduate students in nursing. *Image: Journal of Nursing Scholarship, 31*(3), 289-293.

Kolanko, K. M. (2003). A collective case study of nursing students with learning disabilities. *Nursing Education Perspectives, 23*(5), 251-256.

Kolb, D. (1984). *Experiential learning: Experience as the source of learning and development.* Englewood Cliffs, NJ: Prentice-Hall.

Kuiper, R. (2002). Enhancing metacognition through the reflective use of self-regulated learning strategies. *The Journal of Continuing Education in Nursing, 33*(2), 78-87

Laschinger, H. (1992). Impact of nursing learning environments on adaptive competency development in baccalaureate nursing students. *Journal of Professional Nursing, 8*(2), 105-114.

Lenberg, C. B. (1997). Confusing facets of critical thinking. *Tennessee Nurse, 60*(5), 11, 13.

Linares, A. Z. (1999). Learning styles of students and faculty in selected health care professions. *Journal of Nursing Education, 38*(9), 407-414.

Lipmann, T. H. & Deatrick, J. A. (1997). Preparing advanced practice nurses for clinical decision making in specialty practice. *Nurse Educator, 22*(2), 47-50.

Maheady, D. C. (1999). Jumping through hoops, walking on eggshells: The experiences of nursing students with disabilities. *Journal of Nursing Education, 38*(4), 162-170.

Martin, C. (2002). The theory of critical thinking. *Nursing Education Perspectives, 23*(5), 243-247.

Mayo, K. (1996). Social responsibility in nursing education. *Journal of Holistic Nursing, 14*(1), 24-43.

Moffitt, P. & Wuest, J. (2002). Spirit of the drum: The development of cultural nursing praxis. *Canadian Journal of Nursing Research, 34*(4), 107-116.

Mogale, M., & Botes, A. (2001). Problem-based case study to enhance critical thinking in student nurses. *Curationis: South African Journal of Nursing, 24*(3), 27-35.

Morin, K. (1997). Guest editorial: Critical thinking - Say what? *Journal of Nursing Education, 36*(10), 450-451.

Myrick, F., & Yonge, O. J. (2001). Creating a climate for critical thinking in the preceptorship relationship. *Nurse Educator Today, 21*(6), 461-467.

Myrick, F., & Yonge, O. J. (2004). Enhancing critical thinking in the preceptorship experience in nursing education. *Journal of Advanced Nursing , 45*(4), 371-380.

Nahas, V. (2000). A transcultural study of Jordanian nursing students' care encounters within the context of clinical education. *International Journal of Nursing Studies, 37*(3), 257-266.

Neill, K. M., Lachat, M. F., & Taylor-Panek, S. (1997). Enhancing critical thinking with case studies and nursing process. *Nurse Educator, 22*(2), 30-32.

Oermann, M. H. (1997). Evaluating critical thinking in clinical practice. *Nurse Educator,* 22(5), 25-28.

Ohrling, K., & Hallerg, I. R. (2001). The meaning of preceptorships: Nurses' lived experience of being a preceptor. *Journal of Advanced Nursing, 33*(4), 530-540.

Profetto-McGrath, J., Hesketh, K. L., Lang, S., & Estabrooks, C.A. (2003). A study of critical thinking and research utilization among nurses. *Western Journal of Nursing Research, 25*(3), 322-337.

Rakoczy, M. & Money, S. (1995). Learning styles of nursing students: A 3-year cohort longitudinal study. *Journal of Professional Nursing, 11*(3), 170-174.

Saenz, T., Wyatt, T., & Reinard, J. (1998). Increasing the recruitment and retention of historically underrepresented minority students in higher education: A case study. *American Journal of Speech-Language Pathology, 7*(3), 39-48.

Schell, K. (1998). Promoting student questioning. *Nurse Educator, 23*(5), 8-12.

Schaefer, K. M., & Zygmont, D. (2003). Analyzing the teaching style of nursing faculty: Does it promote a student-center or a teacher-centered learning environment? *Nursing Education Perspectives, 24*(5), 238-245.

Sellappah, S., Hussey, T., Blackmore, A. M., & McMurray, A. (1998). The use of questioning strategies by clinical teachers. *Journal of Advanced Nursing, 28*(1), 142-148.

Simpson, E., & Courtney, M. (2002). Critical thinking in nursing education: Literature review. *International Journal of Nursing Practice, 8*(2), 89-98.

St. Clair, A., & McKenry, L. (1999). Preparing culturally competent practitioners. *Journal of Nursing Education, 38*(5), 228-234.

Tanner, C. (2005). What have we learned about critical thinking in nursing? *Journal of Nursing Education, 44*(2), 47-48.

Thomka, L.A. (2001). Graduate nurses' experiences of interaction with professional nursing staff during transition to the professional role. *The Journal of Continuing Education in Nursing, 32*(1), 15-19.

Thorpe, K., & Loo, R. (2003). The values profile of nursing undergraduate students: Implications for education and professional development. *Journal of Nursing Education, 42*(2), 83-89.

Tsui, L. (2002). Fostering critical thinking through effective pedagogy: Evidence from four institutional case studies. *The Journal of Higher Education, 73*(6), 740-761.

Van Maanen, J., & Schein, E. (1979). Toward a theory of organizational socialization. *Research in Organizational Behavior, 1,* 209-264.

Whiteside, C. (1997). A model for teaching critical thinking in clinical settings. *Dimensions of Critical Care, 16*(3), 152-162.

Wong, U., Kam, F., & Lee, W. M. (2000). A phenomenological study of early nursing experiences in Hong Kong. *Journal of Advanced Nursing, 31*(6), 1509-1517.

Yoder, M. (1996). Instructional responses to ethnically diverse students. *Journal of Nursing Education, 35*(7), 315-321.

Yurovich, E. E. (2001). Working with American Indians toward educational success. *Journal of Nursing Education, 40*(6), 259-269.

CREATING AN EVIDENCE-BASED PRACTICE FOR NURSE EDUCATORS

CHAPTER FOUR
USE ASSESSMENT AND EVALUATION STRATEGIES

A major responsibility of nurse educators is the assessment and evaluation of theoretical and clinical learning. Nurse educators need to be able to conduct formative as well as summative evaluations specifically, and to ensure that methods of evaluation are appropriate to the learning objectives. Educators need to be skilled in item writing, test construction, the use of case studies, group projects, presentations, papers, and a myriad of other ways to assess and evaluate student learning. To use assessment and evaluation strategies effectively the nurse educator:

- Uses extant literature to develop evidence-based assessment and evaluation practices
- Uses a variety of strategies to assess and evaluate learning in the cognitive, psychomotor, and affective domains
- Implements evidence-based assessment and evaluation strategies that are appropriate to the learner and to learning goals
- Uses assessment and evaluation data to enhance the teaching-learning process
- Provides timely, constructive, and thoughtful feedback to learners
- Demonstrates skill in the design and use of tools for assessing clinical practice

Review of Literature

A review of the literature revealed that there are few evidence-based publications related to assessment and evaluation strategies. However, an analysis of what is available led to the identification of four primary themes addressed in the literature: assessment and evaluation of clinical learning, assessment and evaluation of classroom learning, assessment and evaluation of student learning outcomes, and the use of portfolios to assess and evaluate learning.

Assessing and Evaluating Clinical Learning

As noted by Krichbaum, Rowan, Duckett, Ryden, and Savik (1994), the evaluation of clinical performance has been a challenging task for nurse educators throughout our history. Traditionally, clinical performance was based on evaluating the achievement of course objectives. Due to changes in health care practices and nursing education accreditation standards and guidelines, the focus of evaluation has shifted from objectives to outcomes.

Despite its long evolutionary process, the evaluation of clinical performance continues to pose challenges for nurse educators. Krichbaum et al. (1994) provided a comprehensive review of the evolution of clinical evaluation in nursing education and described many of the issues and concerns faced by nursing faculty. One of the major issues regarding clinical evaluation is the lack of uniform standards to evaluate performance and the lack of reliable and valid measurement instruments. In an attempt to address this issue, nurse educators have used a variety of methods and strategies over the past several decades to evaluate students' clinical performance (Gomez, Lobodzinski, & West, 1998), but little empirical evidence exists as to the effectiveness of these methods (Hawranik, 2000).

The evaluation of clinical performance is to some degree influenced by the faculty's perspectives and standards regarding competent performance (Gomez et al., 1998). Goldenberg and Dietrich (2002) described a more humanistic approach to clinical evaluation that emphasizes caring, collaboration, critical thinking, and self-assessment. To minimize the subjectivity and maximize the validity of the evaluation, it is advisable to use multiple evaluation methods.

The literature indicates that the evaluation of clinical performance is enhanced by the use of valid instruments. Bondy, Jenkins, Seymour, Lancaster, and Ishee (1997) developed and tested a valid and reliable measure of psychiatric nursing competencies that could be used with baccalaureate students. Their Psychiatric Nursing Performance Appraisal Instrument (PsychNPAI), which has a coefficient alpha of 0.96, enabled faculty to more clearly articulate performance expectations to students and increased the validity of the clinical evaluation process.

Similarly, Wiles and Bishop (2001) developed and described the use of a graded, criterion-referenced clinical performance appraisal (CPA) to determine clinical grades. The CPA was developed based on Bondy's Criterion Matrix, which enables faculty to rate a student's performance against quantitative as well as qualitative factors and indicate if assistance is required in performing the skill (Bondy et al., 1997). The instrument was subsequently revised after the first semester in use to clarify items and eliminate behaviors that could not be objectively measured (Wiles & Bishop). To strengthen the quality and quantity of feedback provided to students, the CPA was used to rate students after each clinical experience and at the end of each rotation. Students reported that using this instrument helped them be more aware of the criteria for various competencies, provided them with more structured feedback, and improved their performance. Faculty believed that it helped them provide students with a more useful formative evaluation and that use of the ratings motivated students to strive for higher ratings and enhanced the quality of care they provided to patients.

Hawranik (2000) reported on the development and testing of an instrument to measure clinical performance of RN students in a community health course. Using a qualitative approach, students, agency staff, and course faculty were interviewed and/or observed to identify key community health nursing characteristics. These characteristics provided the framework for the instrument, which was used to evaluate student clinical performance. Over a two-year period, the tool was evaluated for clarity, internal consistency, and content validity and was then pilot-tested. Preceptors and students reported that the instrument could be easily completed and it accurately reflected community health nursing practice. The faculty reported that it led to fairer evaluation of students.

Woolley, Bryan, and Davis (1998) described the development of a comprehensive approach to clinical evaluation to reduce subjectivity and bias in evaluation. The components of the comprehensive evaluation plan included professional behaviors; random skill performance; plan of care examination; critical situation examination; and completion of required course assignments that are measured through classroom, on-campus laboratory, and clinical setting observations. Expectations were clearly identified at the beginning of the course. Both faculty and students believe this approach provided a more objective summative evaluation of student performance.

To enhance the clinical evaluation of RN students, Dumas, Villeneuve, and Chevrier (2000) developed an instrument based on Kolb's Experiential Learning Theory (1984) to evaluate the process of clinical learning in RN-BSN students. The instrument provided faculty with formative data related to students' ability to integrate previous experiences with new learning, and it was reported to be a valid and reliable formative evaluation strategy to measure learning.

Wishnia, Yancy, Silva, and Kern-Manwaring (2002) described a unique clinical evaluation approach – evaluation by exception (EBE), which is modeled after the charting by exception method. The purpose for developing this evaluation approach was to make the process of evaluation more efficient and user-friendly. Using this method, the clinical faculty focused the evaluation on "behaviors that deviate from the acceptable standards" (p. 495). Both students and faculty found this method to be more efficient and helpful in guiding future clinical performance. The authors reported that the tool has been shown to be a valid measure of clinical performance. Reliability studies were in the process of being conducted and not reported in this article.

Liberto, Roncher, and Shellenbarger (1999) described the use of anecdotal notes to support clinical evaluation of the student. The authors defined anecdotal notes as brief narrative notations that faculty record regarding observations they make of student behaviors and outcomes while in the clinical setting. While good observational skills are needed to evaluate student performance, it is important for faculty to recall incidents and make conclusions about student performance. Anecdotal notes provide a factual descriptive account of the faculty-student interaction or of the student's observed performance. A comprehensive anecdotal note is one that includes the date of the observation, student name, faculty signature, setting, and description of the student's performance. The authors noted that while the lack of reliability and validity limit the usefulness of anecdotal notes, they serve as a means of documenting clinical performance and provide data for formative and summative evaluation of the student.

Nurse educators have also examined the effectiveness of specific strategies and techniques to enhance performance in the clinical setting. Miller, Nichols, and Beeken (2000) compared videotaped return demonstration and faculty-presented return demonstration for evaluation of clinical skill performance. The evaluation of skill performance did not differ between the two methods. While videotaped return demonstration could decrease faculty evaluation time, it did have some drawbacks, including the observation that it did not make students practice more after viewing the tape to improve performance. The researchers recommended that, regardless of the method used to validate student performance, faculty need to use a consistent approach.

Although journal writing is widely used in nursing education as an evaluation method and has been used as a measure of clinical performance, this evaluation method is not without limitations. Debate exists among nurse educators as to whether or not they should be graded. Holmes (1997) discussed the advantages and disadvantages of grading clinical journals and suggested that there is an incompatibility between the purposes of assigning journal writing (e.g., to encourage self-expression and reflection) and grading journals. Kennison and Misselwitz (2002) conducted a study to examine consistency among faculty in one baccalaureate nursing program in evaluating journals for critical thinking components. Scores given by six faculty were compared to those given by two critical thinking experts. Results indicated that those faculty who described themselves as more abstract thinkers rated the journals higher than those faculty who indicated they were concrete thinkers. Also, faculty who were more familiar with the course concepts tended to rate the journal entries higher. The authors concluded that educators need to "question the process of evaluation for appropriateness, fairness, and consistency" (p. 242).

More recently, the use of concept maps to evaluate clinical judgment and critical thinking skills has been reported in the literature. The use of concept maps has been developed as an alternative to the traditional nursing care plans that have been criticized for being "unrealistic, time consuming … and often copied from books" (Castellino & Schuster, 2002, p. 149). There is some preliminary evidence to suggest that the use of concept maps is an effective method to evaluate the development of critical thinking and clinical judgment skills.

For example, Daley, Shaw, Balistrieri, Glasenapp, and Piacentine (1999) introduced concept maps to 54 senior nursing students enrolled in a clinical course. The maps created by 18 students were randomly selected for data analysis and scoring. A scoring rubric, developed by Novak and Gowin (1984), was used to score the initial and final maps. Based on the rubric, points are awarded for "students' ability to create prepositional links, and analyze and synthesize information" (Daley et al., 1999, pp. 44-45). Two independent scores were obtained for each map to establish reliability ($r = .82$). A comparison of mean scores on first and last maps developed by students showed a significant improvement. In fact, the average score on final maps was 98.16 points higher than the average on first maps, suggesting an increase in conceptual and critical thinking. The authors recommended further research to establish the construct validity of concept maps as a measurement of critical thinking, examine the effectiveness of concept maps with larger samples, and conduct multisite studies.

Castellino and Schuster (2002) compared the effectiveness of clinical concept maps and traditional care plans in promoting critical thinking in 19 RN students in Pakistan. Students developed concepts maps for 17 weeks and, at the end of the term, a survey was completed by faculty and students to evaluate the use of the maps. Although faculty and students reported that the use of concept maps helped students develop a more comprehensive view of the patient's problems and enhance their critical thinking skills, no data are provided to substantiate this conclusion. The authors did not report any scoring procedures for the concept maps nor did they describe any other method of objectively measuring critical thinking.

Another area of research of clinical evaluation methods, particularly in graduate programs, has been the use of standardized patients, individuals who are trained to "realistically and consistently portray a scripted patient role for medical or nursing education or evaluation purposes" (Gibbons et al., 2002, p. 215). In their study, Gibbons et al. used standardized patients along with other teaching strategies, such as skill practice and watching videotapes, to teach and assess 27 graduate nursing students in a health assessment course. Over a five-week time period, the students interacted with various standardized patients in a simulation center. After each session, students were given an opportunity to evaluate their own performance against a checklist and also received feedback from their peers, the patients, and faculty. Using a rating scale, faculty and peers provided feedback on knowledge, organization, and interpersonal skills, while the standardized patients provided feedback on interpersonal skills only. For the final course exam, students videotaped a complete history and physical they performed on a standardized patient. Student course evaluations and final videotaped physical exams skills checklists were used to evaluate the effectiveness of the teaching-learning methods.

Although Gibbons et al. (2002) maintained that the use of standardized patients and other learning methods implemented in this study contributed to higher student satisfaction and final videotaped physical exams that were of much higher quality than those produced by students in a previous class who did not interact with standardized patients, the mean scores on the complete history and physical exams for both classes were essentially the same. The authors also noted that the combination of several teaching-learning strategies (e.g., increased faculty feedback, increased practice time, use of standardized patients) contributed to the effectiveness of the course. While the use of several evaluation methods may have resulted in higher student satisfaction, it did not impact the students' academic achievement as measured by the final videotaped physical exam. In addition, there are methodological issues that need to be considered in evaluating the results of this study. First, there is no indication that inter-rater reliability for the evaluation of student performance was established, and second, it is unknown if any group differences (e.g., GPA, previous course grades) existed between students in the study and students who had previously completed the course.

Other researchers have studied the effectiveness of using standardized patients. Vessey and Huss (2002) determined that the use of standardized patients in a one-time videotaped simulation experience lacked "the necessary reliability and validity to appropriately evaluate clinical skills of nurse practitioner students" (p. 29) in a summative evaluation. Students in this study reported feelings of anxiety related to being videotaped, the lack of nonverbal feedback they received during the experience, and the fact that their clinical grade was dependent upon this one performance. In this study, the performance of students using standardized patients was not reflective of students' performance on certification exams and other clinical evaluation methods. However, it is possible the variables that created anxiety for the students may have impacted the students' performance. The authors recommended that standardized patients be used as a formative evaluation experience and that faculty make multiple visits to clinical sites to accurately evaluate student performance. It can also be stated that it is important for nurse educators to develop competency in the effective use of such simulated evaluation scenarios, whether the scenarios be simulated through the use of standardized patients or high-fidelity simulation technology.

Working with Australian BSN students, Dunn, Stockhausen, Thornton, and Barnard (1995) examined the relationship between selected learning outcomes and the structure of clinical experiences (one day/week for 14 weeks, two days every second week, and a two-week block at end of semester). Findings showed that students preferred the two-week time block because it provided continuity in patient care, increased their self-confidence, enhanced their proficiency in implementing nursing interventions, and enhanced their ability to apply theory to practice. In addition, all students performed significantly better on all measured learning outcomes during the two-week block format than during the 14-week experience. The authors acknowledged factors that may have influenced the study's findings, such as instructor characteristics and variability in clinical settings, but justifiably noted that these factors are not easily controlled in educational research.

Given the significance of clinical practice as a component of nursing education, it was surprising to find the paucity of evidence-based literature to support the various clinical evaluation methods used by nurse educators. Although various methods of clinical evaluation have been described (e.g., journal writing), the effectiveness of these methods has not been empirically tested, nor has the competencies required by faculty to effectively implement these clinical evaluation methods in the curriculum been addressed. During the past decade, few studies have been published reporting on the development and testing of clinical evaluation instruments. As noted in the literature, the evaluation of clinical learning is a complex phenomenon that is affected by many variables, making its measurement a challenge. Nonetheless, faculty are responsible for evaluating students' clinical performance. It is important that more research be conducted to develop and test the validity and reliability of evaluation instruments that faculty use to make such critical decisions, as well as develop an understanding of the competencies required by faculty to effectively evaluate student clinical performance. This is particularly important in light of the fact that much of the clinical teaching in nursing programs is actually the responsibility of part-time clinical faculty who are expert clinicians but may not be academically prepared as nurse educators in evaluation methods.

It should also be noted that, although limited in quantity and scope, the available research is primarily focused on undergraduate nursing education. Recent research focusing on graduate clinical education is limited to the use of standardized patients. Given the proliferation of advanced practice programs, it is equally important to establish valid and reliable instruments to measure clinical performance at the graduate level.

In addition, research focusing on the format of clinical experiences is virtually nonexistent. One way to enhance the evidence base of clinical evaluation is for faculty to share their research, collaborate across institutions, conduct multisite studies, and build upon each others' work rather than conducting small, isolated studies.

Assessing and Evaluating Classroom Learning

The administration of exams is probably the most widely used method to evaluate knowledge gains in nursing students. Educators have used a wide variety of exam formats to evaluate student learning of theoretical content, including multiple-choice, true/false, matching, and essay tests. The use of any type of exam has its advantages and disadvantages (Rasmussen, Speck, & Twigg, 1998). It is interesting to note, however, that while educators rely heavily on exams to measure learning, very little empirical evidence exists on the validity and reliability of various exam formats. Although exams are an efficient and objective way to test knowledge, time and expertise are needed to plan, construct, and administer valid exams that will yield useful data (DeYoung, 2003; Gaberson, 1996; Rasmussen et al., 1998; Tomey, 1999).

The multiple-choice format traditionally has been a popular format for exams. The development of items that measure students' higher-order thinking skills can be a difficult and time-consuming task for educators (Rasmussen et al., 1998). Cross (2000) surveyed a randomly selected sample (N = 66) of baccalaureate and associate degree degree nursing programs in 31 states to determine the types of questions used in exams. Multiple-choice items were the most frequently used items on exams (91.9%), followed by math/calculation questions, matching, true/false, short answers, and essay items. More than half the multiple-choice items were judged by two expert educators to be at the lowest cognitive level and only about 6% were at the two highest levels which would require the application and synthesis of knowledge. Although the study included only a small sample of nursing programs, Cross urged faculty to closely examine the validity of their exams in measuring student learning and, specifically, students' critical thinking abilities.

As an alternative to developing their own exams, some faculty have relied on the use of test banks to measure student learning. Research suggests, however, that these exams may not provide educators with a valid measure of learning. Masters et al. (2001) reviewed test items from 17 test banks and found that many were poorly constructed and the majority (47.3%) of test items was written at the knowledge level of cognitive understanding. In addition, important content related to a topic was not reflected in the test items. The authors recommended that test banks be used with caution and that faculty conduct further research on developing test items. For example, is one type of item stem (e.g., question or sentence completion) more effective than other types in measuring learning outcomes? Does the number of response options for a multiple-choice exam affect test performance? While Masters et al. provided guidelines for writing multiple-choice questions, they acknowledged there is little empirical evidence to support their use.

The use of the essay format provides faculty with an alternative method to assess student learning. Oermann (1999) contends that essay exams "provide a means of assessing higher-level and complex learning outcomes not able to be measured through objective testing" (p. 32). An obvious disadvantage of essay exams is that it is more difficult to score them. However, Oermann offered several techniques that faculty can use as they develop essay exams as well as strategies to reduce bias in grading these exams.

Smith (1996) used poetry to test graduate students' knowledge about physical assessment. A poem, reflecting the attitudes of many geriatric patients, was used in an assessment course. The students responded to a series of open-ended questions dealing with assessment and intervention. The use of poetry appeared to enhance the divergent thinking of students. The authors noted that the students responded positively to this method of testing; however, no data were provided as to its effectiveness in enhancing the students' physical assessment skills.

While exams are generally used to evaluate student learning at the end of a learning experience (e.g., unit exams, final exams), classroom assessment techniques (CATs) provide a means of assessing student progress during the learning experience. Based on this feedback, faculty can revise teaching/learning experiences as needed to enhance student learning outcomes. Perhaps the most frequently referenced work in the area of classroom assessment is that of Angelo and Cross (1993). Several research studies related to the use of CATs were found in the literature.

Eisenbach, Golich, and Curry (1998) reported on the use of CATs across three different courses (political science, management, literature and writing). Pre- and post- surveys were used to assess the students' confidence level about the content at the beginning and end of the course. One-minute papers were used throughout the semester to answer two questions: "What information that we have covered today could have practical applications for you outside the classroom?" and "What was the muddiest point in today's class session?" (p. 61). A mid-semester feedback form was also created to assess students' perceptions of the course. Eisenbach et al. concluded that using CATs provided valuable information regarding student learning, enabled students and faculty to reflect on the learning process, and helped focus the teaching-learning process. Although the authors stated that students in all three courses "reported a much higher level of confidence at the end of the semester" (p. 63), no data were provided to determine if this was a significant difference.

Fitt and Heverly (1994) developed a CAT to assess students' competencies at the beginning of a graduate level research design course in education and social sciences. Students were again asked to rate their perceived competency level at the end of the course. In addition, to validate student ratings, faculty were asked to rate the extent to which each competency was actually covered during the semester. The authors found that this method of assessment helped redirect the teaching as needed, enhanced student participation in learning, and promoted reflection on the learning process for both students and faculty.

While the use of CATs has increased in nursing education, very little empirical evidence exists as to their effectiveness. DeYoung (2003) defined assessment of learning as that which is done "simply to find out what and how well people are learning what we teach, without any intent to give a grade" (p. 259). There are a wide variety of CATs that educators can use to assess learning. For example, many faculty report using the one-minute paper to reflect on questions such as "What was the most important thing learned today?" Faculty can then use this information to identify if students are meeting learning objectives or if instructional changes are needed to enhance learning (DeYoung, 2003; Rowles & Cole, 1998). CATs can also be used to assess students' knowledge about a topic prior to beginning a class or unit of content. However, there is no evidence that the use of one-minute papers helps improve teaching or student learning.

Another strategy that can be used to conduct a formative evaluation of student learning is the use of case studies. Conyers and Ritchie (2001) discussed using case studies as a way to conduct formative evaluation of student learning in Australian BSN students. Students attended a 50-minute lecture that was followed by a two-hour tutorial session in which students worked in small groups on a case study. As students worked on the case study, faculty provided probing questions to promote deeper learning. Each module was then assessed by an in-class case study test that students responded to individually. The use of this method provided students with ongoing feedback as they worked through the case studies (in-class group work), provided them with the ability to ask questions as needed, and provided faculty with formative data on student learning to improve subsequent classroom experiences.

A review of literature indicated that very little research has been conducted to examine the effectiveness of classroom evaluation methods. The lack of evidence supporting the validity and reliability of various exam formats is particularly disturbing as exams are one of the most frequently used methods for evaluating learning. As poor test performance may lead to course failure and program dismissal, it is important that faculty develop and administer exams that are a valid measure of learning objectives.

Although formative classroom evaluation methods, such as the use of CATs, have gained popularity, their use also lacks empirical evidence. Research is needed to determine if use of these strategies enhances students' achievement of learning outcomes.

Assessing and Evaluating Student Learning Outcomes

As a result of changes in accreditation standards that have mandated the documentation of student learning outcomes, a considerable amount of literature can be found describing teaching and evaluation strategies that promote achievement of outcomes. Although formative and summative evaluation strategies have been reported to assess individual students' progress as well as document achievement of program outcomes, the validity and reliability of these measures need to be considered.

Among the various competencies and outcomes described in the literature, critical thinking has perhaps received the most attention. However, despite the plethora of articles that have been published on the topic, the assessment and evaluation of critical thinking continues to be a challenge. Measuring individual students' critical thinking skills was discussed in the competency "Facilitate Learner Development and Socialization" (chapter 3), and the reader is referred to this chapter or the literature related to individual students' critical thinking. In terms of program outcomes, a number of nursing programs have used quantitative measurements such as the California Critical Thinking Skills Test, the California Critical Thinking Disposition Inventory, and the Watson-Glaser Critical Thinking Appraisal to document critical thinking outcomes (McCarthy, Schuster, & Zehr, 1999; Thompson & Rebeschi, 1999; Vaughn-Wrobel, O'Sullivan, & Smith, 1997). Adams, Whitlow, Stover, and Johnson (1996) reviewed four commonly used instruments used to measure critical thinking and summarized the research in which these tools were used. They concluded that although these tools are reliable and valid, the small, convenient samples used in the studies limit generalization of the findings. To maximize the validity of findings, faculty need to consider if the instrument used is appropriate for the nursing curriculum. An important concept for faculty to consider when selecting a standardized measure of critical thinking is that the definition of critical thinking on which the instrument is based must be consistent with the critical thinking definition used within the nursing program. Further research needs to be conducted to document the link between specific critical thinking strategies used in the curriculum and the achievement of program outcomes.

A number of articles have been published that describe methods to promote and evaluate certain expected outcomes of nursing education (e.g., communication skills, critical thinking). The majority of these articles report on teaching and evaluating critical thinking skills of students as they progress through a nursing program. Mastrian and McGonigle (1999) used technology-based active assignments and collaborative learning assignments to promote critical thinking. Critical thinking assignments included the use of electronic email and computer conferencing. Course assignments included critical thinking exercises related to course objectives and World Wide Web assignments. Although the authors felt that the critical thinking skills of students improved, no objective method was used to assess learning outcomes.

Todd (1998) used email to answer challenging, high-level questions as a way to increase critical thinking skills. The method was judged to be valuable despite the challenges of technology. Email provided a means of correcting misinformation and provided an avenue for participation by students who may not actively engage in classroom discussions. This article did not provide any evidence to support the assertion that the use of the Internet or email is an effective method to enhance students' critical thinking skills.

Hiebert (1996) described the use of learning circles as a strategy to increase critical thinking. During each rotation, learning circles consisting of eight participants were scheduled weekly, with the clinical instructor acting as facilitator. These circles were used as a means of closure for the clinical week. Each participant served as a leader and presented a topic for group discussion. The authors felt that learning circles were a cooperative learning technique that facilitated development of critical thinking skills.

Peer review clinical round experiences have also been found to be an effective means of promoting critical thinking (Sedlak & Doheny, 1998). When beginning baccalaureate nursing students (N = 19) led clinical walking rounds in which they presented a patient to the group, responded to questions, and reflected on the care provided, they engaged in active student learning and peer collaboration, which enhanced their critical thinking. The students' critical thinking was assessed by soliciting student feedback about their peer review experiences and noting the affective dimensions of their replies.

Morrison and Free (2001) described the use of multiple-choice test items as a means of measuring critical thinking. The multiple-choice questions were written at the application level or higher, required more than one fact, concept, or construct to answer, and had high discrimination. However, no empirical evidence was presented to support the idea that the use of multiple-choice test items increased the students' ability to think critically.

Youngblood and Beitz (2001) described the use of active learning strategies to develop critical thinking. These included portfolio development, clinical journals, clinical reaction papers, group presentations, case studies, examination analyses, and cooperative learning activities. Unfortunately, the effectiveness of these strategies was not empirically measured, so one cannot comment on their effect on student critical thinking skills or abilities.

Van Eerden (2001) reported on the use of critical thinking vignettes in one ADN program to evaluate student learning of nursing interventions. Vignettes that represented the complexity of nursing care were developed for nursing skills courses, and students were required to successfully perform skills in communication, patient teaching, problem solving, and so on. The author noted that the effectiveness of this teaching strategy in improving clinical performance is under investigation; preliminary data suggest, however, that this is a promising critical thinking evaluation method.

Angel, Duffey, and Belyea (2000) compared the effectiveness of two learning strategies in evaluating students' critical thinking skills. Students completed a health pattern assessment using either a structured format, predetermined by the faculty (N = 72), or an unstructured format, designed by the students (N = 70). While the authors hypothesized that the use of the unstructured method would result in higher critical thinking scores, results showed no significant difference in critical thinking between the two groups.

The measurement of end-of-program outcomes in nursing education is now expected by accrediting agencies; however, the various methods used to measure these outcomes have not been adequately tested through research. As previously noted, a pervasive problem in nursing education research is that much of the existing research reflects small, isolated studies that individually do not have much significance for developing the science of nursing education. It is essential that collaborative efforts among researchers in nursing education be established to design and conduct research that will yield useful knowledge related to the assessment and evaluation of learning and help build the science base for nursing education.

Using Portfolios to Assess Learning

Another theme of assessment and evaluation strategies that was identified in the literature is the use of portfolios. Portfolios, which are collections of the student's work that show growth over time, or collections of the student's best work, have been used to facilitate, assess, and evaluate student learning. For example, Gallagher (2001) used standards-based portfolios (SBP), defined as a "collection of student work that addresses a number of predetermined tasks directly related to the learning outcomes developed for the unit of study" (p. 197), as a means to assess learning and the extent to which students met specific criteria that reflected the learning outcomes. Williams (2001) used portfolios to enhance students' clinical learning. Students were required to document their learning activities related to clinical practice in various sections of the clinical notebook. The notebooks included sections on clinical preparation, professional development, patients' perspectives, and self-awareness. This strategy provided students and faculty with a way to document, assess, and evaluate clinical learning over the course of the semester. Ryan and Carlton (1997) found the portfolio to be an effective tool to document personal and professional progress in academic and professional career development.

Wenzel, Briggs, and Puryear (1998) developed the Integrated Proficiency-Criterion Framework (IPC), based on Benner's Novice-to-Expert model and the National League for Nursing Accrediting Commission's (NLNAC) program outcomes for communication, critical thinking, therapeutic nursing interventions, professional development, personal development, and scholarship. The IPC defines the various competency levels for program outcomes that are expected of the student throughout the program. Students are responsible for selecting appropriate content for their portfolios that reflect the required level criteria. Novice learners are provided with more specific guidelines on how to select content for inclusion in their portfolios. As they progress through the program, students are expected to become more independent in selecting portfolio materials. When students reach the final year in the program, the portfolio provides a synthesis and summative evaluation of their learning. The authors stated that this proposed framework requires testing for use in nursing education.

As documented by Williams (2001), an advantage of using portfolios in clinical learning situations is that it provides faculty with a synthesis of the students' work over the course of a clinical rotation. However, this method may not work as effectively with all students in all situations. McMullan et al. (2003) reviewed the literature on the use of portfolios and summarized the advantages and disadvantages of using this method. Educators have found that the content of portfolios may be influenced by the method of evaluation. For example, if the portfolio is to be graded, students may document "what the instructor wants to hear," rather than their true feelings and experiences, thereby making the portfolio less effective than it could be.

While much has been written about the use of portfolios (Karlowicz, 2000; McMullan et al., 2003; Wenzel et al., 1998), there is very little empirical research on their use and effectiveness. The review of the literature indicated that portfolios have been used as a means of formative as well as summative evaluation in nursing education, but there is a lack of empirical evidence to support their effectiveness. The review conducted by McMullan et al. posed some interesting questions for educators when considering the use of portfolios. If students are just including "what the instructor wants to hear" in their portfolios, is any learning taking place or are students simply engaged in busywork? Research is needed to determine the impact of using portfolios on students' academic achievement.

Identified Gaps in the Literature

A review of the literature indicates that over the past decade there has been a lack of research focused on educator competencies in assessment and evaluation in nursing education. Although educators have developed and used a myriad of evaluation measures for classroom and clinical learning experiences in nursing education, there is a lack of empirical data to demonstrate the appropriateness and effectiveness of these various measures. The majority of articles that were reviewed described how an evaluation strategy was used to measure learning in a particular course or program. Although some of the articles provided anecdotal information on student and faculty satisfaction with the strategy, they did not report data demonstrating impact on learning outcomes. Future research needs to address whether or not a specific assessment or evaluation strategy makes a difference in student learning.

Overall, the evaluation of clinical learning has received more attention in the literature than the evaluation of classroom learning. However, much of the literature on the evaluation of clinical learning is not evidence-based. Furthermore, the focus of existing research has been more on undergraduate education than on graduate education. A review of the literature indicates that the available research is limited in terms of quantity and quality. As noted by Hawranik (2000), the time needed to develop sound measurement instruments may have contributed to the lack of research in this area.

A few researchers in nursing education in the United States and abroad have taken on the challenging task of developing and testing clinical evaluation instruments (e.g., Arthur, 1999; Bondy et al., 1997). Their work provides an excellent basis for replication and/or extension studies. Given the complexity of the practice setting and the demands placed on nursing professionals, it is imperative that nurse educators acquire the competencies required to develop valid and reliable instruments to measure students' performance. It is particularly important to develop evaluation instruments that reflect measurable competencies that can be used to discriminate among levels of students' performance.

In terms of measuring program outcomes, there are a plethora of articles describing assessment and evaluation strategies to measure students' critical thinking skills. Again, much of this literature is not evidence-based. However, there has been some research studies published (e.g., Daley et al., 1999; Castellino & Schuster, 2002) on the use of concept maps to evaluate critical thinking skills that indicates this may be one teaching strategy that enhances students' critical thinking skills. Further work in this area may prove to be very fruitful and provide nurse educators with a more valid measurement of critical thinking.

In addition to the use of concept maps, other strategies have been described in the literature to assess and evaluate end-of-program outcomes, such as the use of reflective journaling and portfolios. The literature indicates that there is debate among nurse educators with respect to the use and grading of journals and portfolios. Research is needed to determine their effectiveness on student learning.

Priorities for Future Research

As indicated at the beginning of this chapter, nurse educators must be able to select, develop, and implement assessment and evaluation strategies that accurately measure student learning and improve the overall teaching-learning process. Currently, very little evidence-based research exists in this area. Based on a review of literature and the competencies identified for nurse educators, the following priorities for research have been identified:

- What are the best practices for evaluating clinical learning in basic and graduate nursing education?

- What is the effect of the use of simulations (e.g., standardized patients and patient simulators) on developing students' clinical competence?

- What are the best practices in the use of journaling and portfolios to evaluate student learning?

- What effect does the use of concept mapping have on students' critical thinking abilities and their ability to synthesize complex information?

- How does the structure of the clinical experience (e.g., number of hours, days, weeks; weekly experiences through a semester vs. concentrated experiences) affect student learning outcomes?

References

Adams, M., Whitlow, J., Stover, L., & Johnson, K. (1996). Critical thinking as an educational outcome. *Nurse Educator, 21*(3), 23-32.

Angel, B., Duffey, M., & Belyea, M. (2000). An evidence-based project for evaluating strategies to improve knowledge acquisition and critical-thinking performance in nursing students. *Journal of Nursing Education, 39*(5), 219-228.

Angelo, T.A., & Cross, P. (1993). *Classroom assessment techniques: A handbook for college teachers* (2nd ed.). Hoboken, NJ: John Wiley & Sons.

Arthur, D. (1999). Assessing nursing students' basic communication and interviewing skills: The development and testing of a rating scale. *Journal of Advanced Nursing, 29*(3), 658-665.

Bondy, K., Jenkins, K., Seymour, L., Lancaster, R., & Ishee, J. (1997). The development and testing of a competency-focused psychiatric nursing clinical evaluation instrument. *Archives of Psychiatric Nursing, 1*(2), 66-73.

Castellino, A., & Schuster, P. (2002). Evaluation of outcomes in nursing students using clinical concept map care plans. *Nurse Educator, 27*(4), 149-150.

Conyers, V., & Ritchie, D. (2001). Case study class tests: Assessment directing learning. *Journal of Nursing Education, 40*(1), 40-42.

Cross, K. W. (2000). *Cognitive levels of multiple-choice items on teacher-made tests in nursing education.* Unpublished dissertation. Wayne State University, UMI No. AAE9992186.

Daley, B., Shaw, C., Balistieri, T., Glasenapp, K., & Piacentine, L. (1999). Concept maps: A strategy to teach and evaluate critical thinking. *Journal of Nursing Education, 38*(1), 42-47.

DeYoung, S. (2003). *Teaching strategies for nurse educators.* Upper Saddle River, NJ: Prentice Hall.

Dumas, L., Villeneuve, J., & Chevrier, J. (2000). A tool to evaluate how to learn from experience in clinical settings. *Journal of Nursing Education 39*(6), 251-258.

Dunn, S. V., Stockhausen, L., Thornton, R., & Barnard, A. (1995). The relationship between clinical education format and selected student learning outcomes. *Journal of Nursing Education, 34*(1), 16-24.

Eisenbach, R., Golich, V., & Curry, R. (1998). Classroom assessment across the disciplines. *New Directions for Teaching and Learning, 73,* 59-66.

Fitt, D., & Heverly, M. (1994). Classroom assessment of student competencies. *Assessment & Evaluation in Higher Education, 19*(3), 215-224.

Gaberson, K. (1996). Test design: Putting all the pieces together. *Nurse Educator, 21*(4), 28-33.

Gallagher, P. (2001). An evaluation of a standards based portfolio. *Nurse Education Today, 21*(3), 197-200.

Gibbons, S., Adamo, G., Padden, D., Ricciardi, R., Graziano, M., Levine, E., & Hawkins, R. (2002). Clinical evaluation in advanced practice nursing education: Using standardized patients in health assessment. *Journal of Nursing Education, 41*(5), 215-221.

Goldenberg, D., & Dietrich, P. (2002). A humanistic-educative approach to evaluation in nursing. *Nurse Education Today, 22*(4), 301-310.

Gomez, D., Lobodzinski, & West, C. (1998). Evaluating clinical performance. In Billings, D. & Halstead, J. (Eds). *Teaching in nursing: A guide for faculty.* Philadelphia: W.B. Saunders.

Hawranik, P. (2000). The development and testing of a community health nursing clinical evaluation tool. *Journal of Nursing Education, 39*(6), 266-272.

Hiebert, J. (1996). Learning circles: A strategy for clinical practicum. *Nurse Educator, 21*(3), 37-42.

Holmes, V. (1997). Grading journals in clinical practice: A delicate issue. *Journal of Nursing Education, 36*(10), 489-492.

Karlowicz, K. (2000). The value of student portfolios to evaluate undergraduate nursing programs. *Nurse Educator, 25*(2), 82-87.

Kennison, M., & Misselwitz, S. (2002). Evaluating reflective writing for appropriateness, fairness, and consistency. *Nursing Education Perspectives, 23* (5), 238-242.

Kolb, D. (1984). *Experiential learning: Experience as the source of learning and development.* Englewood Cliffs, NJ: Prentice-Hall.

Krichbaum, K., Rowan, M., Duckett, L., Ryden, M., & Savik, K. (1994). The clinical evaluation tool: A measure of the quality of clinical performance of baccalaureate nursing students. *Journal of Nursing Education, 33*(9), 395-404.

Liberto, T., Roncher, M., & Shellenbarger, T. (1999). Anecdotal notes: Effective clinical evaluation and record keeping. *Nurse Educator, 24*(6), 15-18.

Masters, J., Husmeyer, B., Pike, M., Leichty, K., Miller, M., & Verst, A. (2001). Assessment of multiple-choice questions in selected test banks accompanying text books used in nursing education. *Journal of Nursing Education, 40*(1), 25-32.

Mastrian, K., & McGonigle, D. (1999). Using technology-based assignments to promote critical thinking. *Nurse Educator, 24*(1), 45-47.

McCarthy, P., Schuster, P., & Zehr, P. (1999). Evaluation of critical thinking in a baccalaureate nursing program. *Journal of Nursing Education, 38*(3), 142-144.

McMullen, M., Endacott, R., Gray, M., Jasper, M., Miller, C., Scholes, J., & Webb, C. (2003). Portfolios and assessment of competence: A review of the literature. *Journal of Advanced Nursing, 41*(3), 283-294.

Melland, H., & Volden, C. (1998). Classroom assessment: Linking teaching and learning. *Journal of Nursing Education, 37*(6), 275-277.

Miller, H., Nichols, E., & Beeken, J. (2000). Comparing videotaped and faculty-present return demonstrations of clinical skills. *Journal of Nursing Education, 39*(5), 237-239.

Morrison, S., & Free, K. (2001). Writing multiple-choice test items that promote and measure critical thinking. *Journal of Nursing Education, 40*(1), 17-24.

Nieswiadomy, R. M., Arnold, W. K., & Garza, C. (2001). Changing answers on multiple-choice examinations taken by baccalaureate nursing students. *Journal of Nursing Education, 40*(3), 142-144.

Novak, J., & Gowin, D. B. (1984). *Learning how to learn.* New York: Cambridge Press.

Oermann, M. (1999). Developing and scoring essay tests. *Nurse Educator, 24*(2), 29-32.

Rasmussen, L., Speck, D. & Twigg, P. (1998). Developing and using classroom tests. In Billings, D. & Halstead, J. (Eds). *Teaching in nursing: A guide for faculty* (pp. 385-405). Philadelphia: W.B. Saunders.

Rowles, C. J., & Cole, P. J. (1998). Improving teaching and learning: Classroom assessment techniques. In D. M. Billings & J. A. Halstead (Eds.), *Teaching in nursing: A guide for faculty* (pp. 275 -280). Philadelphia: W.B. Saunders.

Ryan, M., & Carlton, K. H. (1997). Portfolio applications in a school of nursing. *Nurse Educator, 22*(1), 35-39.

Sedlak, C., & Doheny, M. (1998). Peer review through clinical rounds: A collaborative critical thinking strategy. *Nurse Educator, 23*(5), 42-45.

Shelton, E. (2003). Faculty support and student retention. *Journal of Nursing Education, 42*(2), 68-76.

Smith, M. (1996). The use of poetry to test nursing knowledge. *Nurse Educator, 21*(5), 20-22.

Thompson, C. & Rebeschi, L. (1999). Critical thinking skills of baccalaureate nursing students at program entry and exit. *Nursing & Health Care Perspectives, 20*(5), 248-252.

Todd, N. (1998). Using e-mail in an undergraduate nursing course to increase critical thinking skills. *Computers in Nursing, 16*(2), 115-118.

Tomey, A. (1999). Selected response test item. *Nurse Educator, 24*(5), 9-13.

Van Eerden, K. (2001). Using critical thinking vignettes to evaluate student learning. *Nursing & Health Care Perspectives, 22*(5), 231-234.

Vaughan-Wroebel, B., O'Sullivan, P., & Smith, L. (1997). Evaluating critical thinking skills of baccalaureate nursing students. *Journal of Nursing Education, 36*(10), 485-488.

Vessey, J., & Huss, K. (2002). Using standardized patients in advanced practice nursing education. *Journal of Professional Nursing, 18*(1), 29-35.

Wenzel, L., Briggs, K., & Puryear, B. (1998). Portfolio: Authentic assessment in the age of the curriculum revolution. *Journal of Nursing Education, 37*(5), 208-212.

Wiles, L., & Bishop, J. (2001). Clinical performance appraisal: Renewing graded clinical experiences. *Journal of Nursing Education, 40*(1), 37-39.

Williams, J. (2001). The clinical notebook: Using student portfolios to enhance clinical teaching learning. *Journal of Nursing Education, 40*(3), 135-137.

Wishnia, G., Yancy, P., Silva, J., & Kern-Manwaring, N. (2002). Evaluation by exception for nursing students. *Journal of Nursing Education, 41*(11), 495-497.

Woolley, G., Bryan., M., & Davis, J. (1998). A comprehensive approach to clinical evaluation. *Journal of Nursing Education, 37*(8), 361-366.

Youngblood, N., & Beitz, J. (2001). Developing critical thinking with active learning strategies. *Nurse Educator, 26*(1), 39-42.

CREATING AN EVIDENCE-BASED PRACTICE FOR NURSE EDUCATORS

CHAPTER FIVE
PARTICIPATE IN CURRICULUM DESIGN AND EVALUATION OF PROGRAM OUTCOMES

Nurse educators need to be knowledgeable about the process of curriculum design and evaluation of program outcomes. It is important for educators to think of the curriculum as a dynamic process that provides a broad framework for a program, yet is flexible enough to change as needed to meet discipline, community, and societal needs. It is critical that all faculty understand the curriculum as an integrated whole, as well as how their particular courses and areas of expertise fit in and contribute to the larger curriculum design. Educators must understand, for example, the prerequisites needed as a basis for their courses and how meeting the objectives of one course allows students to build upon that knowledge in subsequent learning experiences. Armed with such understanding, faculty will be better prepared to make sound decisions about designing curricula, making curriculum revisions, selecting teaching methodologies, and determining evaluation strategies.

To effectively participate in curriculum design and evaluation of program outcomes, the nurse educator:

- Ensures that the curriculum reflects institutional philosophy and mission, current nursing and health care trends, and community and societal needs, so as to prepare graduates for practice in a complex, dynamic, multicultural health care environment
- Demonstrates knowledge of curriculum development, including identifying program outcomes, developing competency statements, writing learning objectives, and selecting appropriate learning activities and evaluation strategies
- Bases curriculum design and implementation decisions on sound educational principles, theory, and research
- Revises the curriculum based on assessment of program outcomes, learner needs, and societal and health care trends
- Implements curricular revisions using appropriate change theories and strategies
- Creates and maintains community and clinical partnerships that support educational goals
- Collaborates with external constituencies throughout the process of curriculum revision
- Designs and implements program assessment models that promote continuous quality improvement in all aspects of the program

Review of the Literature

It is interesting to note that research articles focusing on faculty competencies in curriculum design and program evaluation were limited. When information specific to the concept of "curriculum competency" was found to be rather limited, additional investigation was conducted searching for the terms "curriculum evaluation" and "program evaluation." After gaps in this review were identified, additional references with a logical fit were sought to complete the review.

The literature in general identifies and discusses the need for curriculum change, reports survey data on recommended curricular content, and describes case examples of curriculum projects (both content and process approaches). Case reports account for the majority of articles in this review. Some survey data were reported, with limited research data beyond this. Specific themes in the literature relevant to this competency included: recommended curriculum content specific to health care trends/societal needs; curriculum development activities; adapting teaching/learning methods to meet changing needs; encouraging faculty development to engage in curriculum design activities; accreditation issues and professional standards; competency-based programs; and curriculum/program evaluation. A summary of literature relevant to this competency, and organized around the identified themes, follows.

Addressing Health Care Trends and Societal Needs in the Curriculum

Many articles reviewed for this analysis were commentaries or survey reports of recommended curricular content based on changing societal needs, evolution of health care, and changes in the health care system. For example, topics discussed by authors as necessary additions to curriculum included gerontology (Yurchuck & Brower, 1994); genetics (Prows et al., 2003); managed care (Brzytwa, Copeland, & Hewson, 2000); complementary health (Richardson, 2003); violence prevention, assessment, and treatment (Woodtli & Breslin, 2002); transcultural concepts and faculty preparedness to teach these concepts (Ryan, Carlton, & Ali, 2000); and leadership and management (Meeker & Byers, 2003). Callister, Bond, Matsumura, and Mangum (2004) reported, in their survey of 132 baccalaureate nursing programs, that there was a lack of content related to spiritual nursing care. On a broader scope, Gubrud-Howe et al. (2003) described a statewide effort to help shape nursing education in Oregon, including needed curriculum change and plans for implementing such changes.

Discussions of curriculum needs regarding community health or primary care were more numerous, reflecting the emphasis on community-based care that had developed in health care in the previous decade. Shoultz and Amundson (1998) commented on the need for a nursing curriculum focused on community-based primary health care, addressing the need for nurses to stay current with the changing health care system. Rationale and process for changing from an acute care to a primary care focused curriculum were offered by Mawn and Reece (2000), and case examples of community-based curriculum implementation were described by several authors (McCahon, Niles, George, & Stricklin, 1999; Conger, Baldwin, Abegglen, & Callister, 1999). Strategies for developing a combined master's program that allowed specialization in community health nursing, nursing administration or nursing informatics tracks were reported in the literature (Westmoreland & Hays, 2002), and descriptions of advanced practice programs that offer a combined community/public health nursing master's and promote development of graduates with leadership competencies in these areas were offered (Kaiser, Barr, & Hays, 2003).

While many of these articles addressed important health care trends and societal needs, it must be noted that the majority of the curriculum revisions described by these authors were not evidence-based. The continuing focus upon content in our nursing education programs, without any evidence that such a focus improves the quality of our graduates and provides them with the competencies they need for contemporary nursing practice, leads to much frustration on the part of teachers and students alike.

Engaging in Curriculum Development Activities

The articles on engaging in curriculum development activities generally focused on two topical areas: conducting needs assessments to guide curriculum revision and selecting strategies to facilitate curriculum development. The use of a "needs assessment" to gain feedback from stakeholders and guide the development of new curricula has been described in several articles. Responding to emerging health care reform in Hong Kong, Tiwari, Chan, and Law (2002) described the importance of involving stakeholders, such as students, health care providers, and policy makers, in determining the need for specific content within the nursing curriculum. They used focus group and individual interviews, workshops, and analysis of documents to gather data to identify the knowledge and skills required for graduate nursing education in Hong Kong as a result of health care reform. They reported this approach to curriculum development to be effective in reflecting the needs of the health care system, practicing nurses, and students. However, they suggested that this approach may result in a short-term view of health care needs and also indicated that questions may arise about the validity of the stakeholders' opinions.

A report from British Columbia identified the use of a Delphi survey to include practicing nurses' perspectives of needed curriculum development (Beddome et al., 1995). A strategy for surveying stakeholders, in this instance nurse managers, was shared by Russell and Scoble (2003).They provided survey results and the final model curriculum that was developed for a graduate nursing management program from the input of 115 nurse managers who responded to their survey.

Gagan, Berg, and Root (2002) addressed maintaining currency of a nurse practitioner curriculum in a changing world and suggested a specific model to assess graduates' abilities within the context of changing communities. Freeman, Voignier, and Scott (2002) provided examples and suggested strategies for developing programs that consider the needs of future graduates in an attempt to keep pace with changing community needs. These strategies included requiring knowledge of basic nursing skills prior to admission to the program, focusing on life skills and technology skills within the curriculum, and emphasizing active learning. Evaluation data from the suggested curricular changes was in the process of being collected, thus no data-based outcomes were reported.

Implications for periodic reevaluation and curriculum adaptation due to a curriculum's short lifespan in the rapidly changing world of health care were discussed and strategies for faculty consensus building and prioritizing were described by Arthur and Baumann (1996). They used a combination of quantitative and qualitative methodologies to focus on core content selection for nursing curricula. Heinrich, Karner, Gaglione, and Lambert (2002) shared tools, including a matrix, to promote visual representation of curricular concepts and concept relationships/implementation within courses.

Kooker, Shoultz, Sloat, and Trotter (1998) described a process for using community-based focus groups as a curriculum development strategy. They reported that, while resource intensive, the use of focus group methodology was effective in providing rich feedback that could be used to develop community-based nursing curricula. Vilakazi, Chabeli, and Roos (2000) described the use of focus groups to determine guidelines and strategies for integrating primary care concepts into a community health course.

Adapting Teaching/Learning Methods to Meet Changing Needs

Several articles reported on how faculty in individual nursing programs were adapting their teaching methodologies to meet changing curricular needs. Strategies for implementing a problem-based learning approach in the curriculum were described by Alexander, McDaniel, Baldwin and Money (2002) in a report on the outcomes of a project that implemented problem-based learning (PBL) into an undergraduate nursing curriculum. They stated that PBL had a positive effect on students as measured by very positive NCLEX results for the program. Morales-Mann and Kaitell (2001) described the implementation of PBL in a Canadian school of nursing. They also reported that the use of PBL was effective; however, they found that students initially were not prepared to participate in PBL and that faculty would also benefit from more training in how to teach using the PBL approach. They recommended increased preparation for both groups to maximize the effectiveness of the teaching strategy.

DeSimone (1996) shared a case report of strategies used to implement transformative leadership competencies into a baccalaureate nursing leadership course. Prior to beginning the course, students and faculty completed a Leadership Performance Competence Profile. Results indicated that students viewed faculty to be competent in leadership performance; faculty viewed students as not competent in leadership performance. Using the Spearman Brown prophecy formula, a reliability of .63 was established for the instrument. Based upon findings from the profile instrument, interactive teaching strategies that fostered communication, decision-making, and a democratic learning environment were incorporated into the course. These strategies included group problem-solving, simulated patient management activities, and evaluation of peers' leadership behaviors. The students also engaged in a 15-week clinical experience that focused on developing leadership competencies. At the end of the course, the instrument was administered again to students and faculty with the results indicating that students' leadership competencies had improved. To what extent these changes were related to the interactive teaching strategies in the classroom or the 15-week clinical experience was difficult to determine.

Eckhardt, Anderson, Campbell and Pavlish (2002) described a framework for developing a reflective practitioner in an RN-to-BSN program. Schreiber and Banister (2002) described a curriculum focused on providing learning opportunities for student dialogue and critical reflection. Ironside (2004) described a study in which she used Heideggerian hermeneutics to explore how the use of new interpretive pedagogies influenced the thinking of faculty. A theme that emerged from this study was that of the relationship between thinking and covering content, and that the use of interpretative pedagogies may help faculty deemphasize the focus on content and place more focus on teaching thinking.

Finally, Ryan, Twibell, Miller, and Brigham (1996) shared a case example of barriers and strategies to promote incorporation of multicultural content through regional networking among nursing schools. The barriers included lack of faculty commitment and knowledge related to cultural diversity content, difficulty and costs associated with establishing cultural clinical experiences, and difficulty integrating cross-cultural concepts throughout the curriculum. Strategies to overcome these barriers included strengthening the school mission to provide cross-cultural experiences, mentoring faculty to increase their competence, seeking funding and shared learning experiences with other departments and schools to decrease costs, and developing program outcomes that address cultural diversity.

Encouraging Faculty Development for Curriculum Revision

Challenges and difficulties in revising or changing curriculum were noted in the literature. Hull, St. Romain, Alexander, Schaff, and Jones (2001) discussed the concept of changing curriculum as being similar to "moving cemeteries." They referred to the use of a six-component collaborative research framework (commitment, compatibility, communication, contribution, consensus, and credit), which they believed helped change their faculties' attitude about curriculum revision.

Many articles addressed the need for faculty development in making decisions about curriculum revision, including the addition and deletion of content. For example, Yurchuck and Brower (1994) described concerns about the lack of faculty preparation in geriatrics and described a strategy for faculty development to teach this specialty. In order to integrate substance abuse topics into the curriculum, Marcus (1997) described strategies including independent learning, consultations, workshops, seminars, and retreats as methods used to update faculty. Chrisman (1998) used faculty seminars, videos, and printed teaching materials as resources to update faculty on strategies for integrating cultural and social diversity concepts into the curriculum. Summer institutes, planned follow-up, and continuing education classes were strategies described by Prows et al. (2003) to both increase faculty knowledge on a new topic and encourage inclusion of genetics in basic nursing programs. Halstead and Coudret (2000) described web-based education and the need for faculty development to promote effective, efficient use of this technology, providing a case example of a web-based RN-to-BSN program implementation.

Diekelmann (2002) described dilemmas of excess curriculum content and faculty tendencies to cling to long-standing approaches to curriculum. She suggested that the new phenomenological pedagogies may help address this issue. Porter-O'Grady (2001) presented challenges for nursing leadership in coping with the rapid changes in the health care environment and the need to prepare nursing students for tomorrow's challenges. Addressing the need for "forecasting" appropriate curricular change, he emphasized that creating a viable future depended on meeting emerging societal needs.

There were a few articles in the literature that addressed how to prepare nurse educators to teach and develop curriculum. Hakkarainen and Janhonen (1997) described a qualitative study of groups of students within an educator course in Finland and their approaches/strategies for developing a variety of undergraduate nursing courses. They recommended revamping teacher education in Finland to better address the developmental needs of nurse teachers. Specific to initiating a nurse educator program in South Africa, Kyriacos and Van Den Heever (1999) described approaches to developing a nontraditional curriculum, including integrating the concepts of flexibility and creativity to meet diverse learner needs. The program was based upon adult education principles and encouraged cooperative learning and interactive teaching strategies. It was evident from these two articles that, internationally, the curriculum of nurse educator programs is undergoing significant revision.

Attending to Accreditation Issues and Professional Standards

The National League for Nursing Accrediting Commission (NLNAC) (2002) and the Commission on Collegiate Nursing Education (CCNE) (1998), as well as other professional organizations, have provided standards and guidelines for curriculum direction. Several articles described the efforts of individual programs of nursing in using professional guidelines and standards to develop curriculum.

In a history and review of the concepts of nurse licensure, accreditation, and certification, Barnum (1997) related these concepts to accreditation issues for nursing schools. She questioned the amount of time that nursing faculty devote to pursuing accreditation and the benefits of professional education accreditation.

Daggett, Butts, and Smith (2002) described curriculum development efforts aimed at achieving a contemporary nursing skill set that was based on the American Association of Colleges of Nursing guidelines for nursing education and addressed the benefits of using such an organizing framework to guide curriculum implementation. Wenzel, Briggs, and Puryear (1998) described an integrated, criterion-based framework that was developed, based upon the NLNAC accreditation criteria and Benner's (1984) model as applied to student proficiency stages. This framework, which they named the Integrated Proficiency-Criterion Framework, was used to develop a portfolio assessement strategy to document student learning of critical thinking, communication, professional development, personal development, therapeutic nursing interventions, and scholarship. Van Ort and Townsend (2002) described the relevance of CCNE standards, programs, and curricula with a community-based nursing focus.

Designing Competency-Based Programs

An increased focus on outcomes assessment has evolved from issues of accountability, and this has led to growth in competency-based education in nursing. Lenburg (2002) provided an overview, context, and rationale for competency-based education and practice, describing selected methods of performance assessment. Redman, Lenburg, and Walker (1999) described one school's implementation of a competency-based curriculum, including assessment strategies designed to accurately document competence in the current practice environment. The process used by faculty to implement a competency-oriented learning approach in the curriculum was described, with emphasis on community-focused primary health care and the creation of interdisciplinary task groups (Perkins, Vale, & Graham, 2001).

Thompson and Bartels (1999) reviewed the literature and identified strategies and guidelines for nurse faculty to establish best practices in outcomes assessment for nursing education. These strategies included gaining faculty and student support for the efforts, identifying assessment methods, and using the assessment results to improve student learning. Forker and Yurchuck (1996) explored the concept of assessment in helping determine competencies for community-based nursing education outcomes. Medical schools provided a large-scale example of competency-based curricular change (Accreditation Council for Graduate Medical Education, 2001).

Evaluating Program Outcomes to Enusre Continuous Quality Improvement

Hamner and Bentley (2003) described a faculty workshop that was used to initiate a new program evaluation plan that included definition of terms, clarification of outcomes, specifications of evaluation methods, means for collecting, analyzing, and trending data, and a mechanism to use findings for further program development. Seager and Anema (2003) discussed the use of Stufflebeam's Model (context, input, process, and product) to facilitate multisite evaluation of an associate degree curriculum. They found the model to be effective in guiding the evaluation of curriculum. Yearwood, Singleton, Feldman, and Colombraro (2001) reported a case study of their use of the continuous quality improvement process and an annual school "report card" evaluating and using program feedback to address major school components ranging from faculty performance to curriculum development and organizational change. This approach was effective in helping faculty take ownership in making decisions about curriculum and organizational change.

In an ex post facto study of 278 baccalaureate nursing students to identify variables that predicted program success (as measured by NCLEX pass rates) Byrd, Garza, and Nieswiadomy (1999) noted the importance of considering admission and progression criteria, along with student demographic variables. In this particular study sample, age, ethnicity, prenursing GPA, and science GPA predicted success in 77% of the students.

Using student portfolios to document student outcomes and demonstrate curriculum effectiveness was described as one method of curriculum evaluation (Martin, Kinnick, Hummel, Clukey, & Baird, 1997; Ramey & Hay, 2003). An emerging concept in program evaluation is that of benchmarking. Billings, Connors, and Skiba (2001) used findings from research in higher education to develop a framework and process for benchmarking best practices in teaching/learning approaches for web-based nursing courses.

Identified Gaps in the Literature

The articles reviewed for this analysis indicated that most of what we know about educators' competency in curriculum design and program evaluation is limited primarily to anecdotal evidence. The curriculum textbooks that were reviewed addressed content relevant to the curriculum and program evaluation competency more so than did articles.   Limited work has been done on identifying specific faculty competencies in curriculum and program evaluation in general.

DeNeef (2002), in describing the Preparing Future Faculty program, emphasized that higher education is not doing a good job of socializing students into educator roles, including the role of participant or leader in curriculum innovations, and limited information exists about strategies for teaching students and novice faculty how to participate effectively in curriculum decisions. More information is needed on best practices for teaching basic skills, such as course development within the context of an overall curriculum, as well as developing teaching strategies and evaluation tools that "fit" with outcomes and competencies for courses and programs.

In addition, the fundamentals of making curriculum decisions in a rapidly changing world with limited time and resources have not been adequately addressed in the literature. Discussion of strategies for coping effectively with challenges such as time and logistics could prove useful, as would analysis of the cost resource allocation issues associated with frequent curricular changes. While there were beginning discussions of web-based learning and program outcomes, integration of such approaches and their impact on overall curriculum design need additional attention.

At a time when focus is on accountability and outcomes of all programs, there is a surprisingly limited discussion of program outcomes and program evaluation methods. Future discussion is needed in these areas as both the nursing profession and broader society call for clarification of outcomes in all types of nursing programs.

Priorities for Future Research

The following questions are offered to stimulate research that will enhance our understanding of the nurse educator competency of designing curricula and evaluating program outcomes:

- What are the elements of curriculum design and program evaluation that are most essential for faculty to master?

- What are the best practices for attaining educator competencies in curriculum design and program evaluation?

- What are the relationships between teaching and learning competencies and competencies in curriculum design and program evaluation?

- What are the best strategies to help graduate students make the transition from clinician to educator as those roles relate to curriculum and program evaluation?

- What are the best practices and benchmark indicators for educator program accountability and effectiveness in preparing students in this competency?
- What are the best models for educational program partnering for effective, efficient program evaluation and curriculum development?
- What are the best models for utilizing program evaluation data to ensure continuous quality improvement within the curriculum?

References

Accreditation Council for Graduate Medical Education (2001). Accreditation Council for Graduate Medical Education Outcome Project. Retrieved from http://www.acgme.org/outcome/project/proHome.asp

Alexander, J.G., McDaniel, G.S., Baldwin, M.S., & Money, B.J. (2002). Promoting, applying, and evaluating problem-based learning in the undergraduate nursing curriculum. *Nursing Education Perspectives, 23*(5), 248-253.

Arthur, H., & Baumann, A. (1996). Nursing curriculum content: An innovative decision-making process to define priorities. *Nurse Education Today, 16*(1), 63-68.

Barnum, B.S. (1997). Licensure, certification, and accreditation online. *Journal of Issues in Nursing.* Retrieved from http://www.nursingworld.org/ojin/tpc4/tpc4_2.htm

Beddome, G., Budgen, C., Hills, M.D., Lindsey, A.E., Duval, P.M., & Szalay, L. J. (1995). Education and practice collaboration: A strategy for curriculum development. *Nurse Educator, 34*(1), 11-15.

Benner, P. E. (1984). *From novice to expert: Excellence and power in clinical nursing practice.* Englewood Cliffs, NJ: Prentice Hall.

Billings, D. M., Connors, H. R., & Skiba, D. J. (2001). Benchmarking best practices in Web-based nursing courses. *Advances in Nursing Science, 23*(3), 41-52.

Brzytwa, E., Copeland, L., & Hewson, M. (2000). Managed care education: A needs assessment of employers and educators of nurses. *Journal of Nursing Education, 39*(5), 197-204.

Byrd, G., Garza, C., & Nieswiadomy, R. (1999). Predictors of successful completion of a baccalaureate nursing program. *Nurse Educator, 24*(6), 33-37.

Callister, L., Bond, A., Matsumura, G., & Mangum, S. (2004). Threading spirituality throughout nursing education. *Holisitic Nursing Practice, 18*(3), 160-166.

Chrisman, N. J. (1998). Faculty infrastructure for cultural competence education. *Journal of Nursing Education, 37*(1), 45-47.

Conger, C. O., Baldwin, J. H., Abegglen, J., & Callister, L. C. (1999). The shifting sands of health care delivery: Curriculum revision and integration of community health nursing. *Journal of Nursing Education, 38*(7), 304-311.

Commission on Collegiate Nursing Education. (1998). *Standards.* Retrieved from http://www.aacn.nche.edu/Accreditation/standrds.htm

Daggett, L. M, Butts, J. B, & Smith, K. K. (2002). The development of an organizing framework to implement AACN guidelines for nursing education. *Journal of Nursing Education, 41,*(1), 34-37.

DeNeef, A. (2002). The Preparing Future Faculty Program: What difference does it make? Washington, DC: Association of American Colleges and Universities.

DeSimone, B. B. (1996). Transforming curriculum for a nursing leadership course: A collaborative approach. *Journal of Professional Nursing, 12*(2), 111-118.

Diekelmann, N. (2002). "Too much content...:" Epistemologies' grasp and nursing education. *Journal of Nursing Education, 41*(11), 469-470.

Eckhardt, J.A., Anderson, D.M., Campbell, S. E., & Pavlish, C.L. (2002). A theoretical framework for RN-to -BSN education. *Nursing Education Perspectives, 23*(3), 124–127.

Fealy, G. (2002). Aspects of curriculum policy in preregistration nursing education in the Republic of Ireland: Issues and reflections. *Journal of Advanced Nursing, 37*(6), 558-565.

Forker, J. E., & Yurchuck, E. R. (1996). Assessing outcomes of community-based nursing education. *Nurse Educator, 21*(2), 15-16.

Freeman, L. H., Voignier, R. R., & Scott, D. L. (2002). New curriculum for a new century: Beyond repackaging. *Journal of Nursing Education, 41*(1), 38-40.

Gagan, M. J., Berg, J., & Root, S. (2002). Nurse practitioner curriculum for the 21st century: A model for evaluation and revision. *Journal of Nursing Education, 41*(5), 202-206.

Gubrud-Howe P, Shaver, K.S., Tanner, C.A., Bennett-Stillmaker, J., Davidson, S.B., Flaherty-Robb, M., Goudreau, K., Hardham, L., Hayden, C., Hendy, S., Omel, S., Potempa, K., Shores, L., Theis, S., & Wheeler, P. (2003). A challenge to meet the future: Nursing education in Oregon 2010. *Journal of Nursing Education, 42*(4), 163–167.

Hakkarainen, P.E., & Janhonen, S. (1997). Teaching practice as a testbench of learning in master's degree education for nurse teachers in Finland. *Nurse Educator Today, 17*(5), 454-462.

Halstead, J.A., & Coudret, N. A. (2000). Implementing Web-based instruction in a school of nursing: Implications for faculty and students. *Journal of Professional Nursing, 16*(5), 273-281.

Heinrich, C.R., Karner, K.J., Gaglione, B.H., & Lambert, L.J. (2002). Order out of chaos: The use of a matrix to validate curriculum integrity. *Nurse Educator, 27*(3), 136-140.

Hamner, J.B., & Bentley, R.W. (2003). A systematic evaluation plan that works. *Nurse Educator, 28*(4), 179-184.

Hiraki, A. (1992). Tradition, rationality, and power in introductory nursing textbooks: A critical hermeneutics study. *Advances in Nursing Scence, 14*(3), 1-12.

Hull, E., St. Romain, J.A., Alexander, P., Schaff, S., & Jones, W. (2001). Moving cemeteries: A framework for facilitating curriculum revision. *Nurse Educator, 26*(6), 280-282.

Ironside, P. (2004). Covering the content and teaching thinking: Deconstructing the additive curriculum. *Journal of Nursing Education, 43*(1), 5-12.

Kaiser, K.L., Barr, K.L., & Hays, B.J. (2003). Setting a new course for advanced practice community/public health nursing. *Journal of Professional Nursing, 19*(4),189-96.

Kooker, B.M., Shoultz, J., Sloat, A.R., & Trotter, C. M. (1998). Focus groups: A unique approach to curriculum development. *Nursing and Health Care Perspectives, 19*(6), 283-286.

Kyriacos, U., & Van Den Heever, J. (1999). A nontraditional curriculum for the preparation of nurse educators. *Journal of Nursing Education, 38*(7), 319-324.

Lenburg, C. (2002). Changes that challenge nursing education. *Tennessee Nurse, 65*(5), 10-13.

Luttrell, M. F., Lenburg, C.B., Scherubel, J.C., Jacob, S.R., & Koch, R. W. (1999). Competency outcomes for learning and performance assessment. Redesigning a BSN curriculum. *Nursing and Health Care Perspectives, 20*(3), 134-141.

Marcus, M.T. (1997). Faculty development and curricular change: A process and outcomes model for substance abuse education. *Journal of Professional Nursing, 13*(3), 168-177.

Martin, J.H., Kinnick, V.L., Hummel, F., Clukey, L., & Baird, S.C. (1997). Developing outcome assessment methods. *Nurse Educator, 22*(6), 35-40.

Mawn, B., & Reece, S.M. (2000). Reconfiguring a curriculum for the new millennium: The process of change. *Journal of Nursing Education, 39*(3), 101-108.

McCahon, C.P., Niles, S.A., George, V.D., & Stricklin, M.L. (1999). A model to restructure nursing education: Vision on 22nd street. *Nursing and Health Care Perspectives, 20*(6), 296-301.

Meeker, P.B., & Byers, J.F. (2003). Data-driven graduate curriculum redesign: A case study. *Journal of Nursing Education, 42*(4),186-188.

Morales-Mann, E.T., & Kaitell, C.A.(2001). Problem-based learning in a new Canadian curriculum. *Journal of Advanced Nursing, 33*(1), 13-19.

National League for Nursing Accrediting Commission (2002). *Accreditation manual & interpretive guidelines by program type.* Retrieved from http://www.nlnac.org/

Perkins, I., Vale, D.J., & Graham, M.S. (2001). Partnerships in primary health care: A process for re-visioning nursing education. *Nursing Health Care Perspectives, 22*(1), 20-25.

Porter-O'Grady, T. (2001). Profound change: 21st century nursing. *Nursing Outlook, 49*(4), 182–186.

Prows, C. A., Hetteberg, C. J., Johnson, N., Latta, K., Lovell, A., Saal, H.M., & Warren, N. S. (2003). Outcomes of a genetics education program for nursing faculty. *Nursing Education Perspectives, 24*(2), 81–85.

Ramey, S.L., & Hay, M.L. (2003). Using electronic portfolios to measure student achievement and assess curricular integrity. *Nurse Educator, 28*(1), 31-36.

Redman, R., Lenburg, C., & Walker, P. (1999). Competency assessment: Methods for development and implementation in nursing education. *Online Journal of Issues of Nursing,* September 30, 12 pp.

Richardson, S. F. (2003). Complementary health and healing in nursing education. *Journal of Holistic Nursing, 21*(1), 20-35.

Russell, G., & Scoble, K. (2003). Vision 2020, part 2: Educational preparation for the future nurse manager. *Journal of Nursing Administration, 33*(7-8), 404-409.

Ryan, M., Carlton, K.H., & Ali, N. (2000). Transcultural nursing concepts and experiences in nursing curricula. *Journal of Transcultural Nursing,11*(4), 300-307.

Ryan, M., Twibell, R., Miller, A., & Brigham, C. (1996). Cross-cultural nursing. A report of faculty collaboration through regional networking. *Nurse Educator, 21*(6), 28-32.

Schreiber, R., & Banister, E. (2002). Challenges of teaching in an emancipatory curriculum. *Journal of Nursing Education, 41*(1), 41-45.

Seager, S., & Anema M. G. (2003). Curriculum issues: A process for conducting a curriculum audit. *Nurse Educator, 28* (1), 5-6.

Shoultz, J., & Amundson, M. J. (1998). Nurse educators' knowledge of primary health care: Implications for community-based education, practice, and research. *Nursing and Health Care Perspectives, 19*(3), 114-119.

Thompson, C., & Bartels, J. E. (1999). Outcomes assessment: Implications for nursing education. *Journal of Professional Nursing, 15*(3), 170-178.

Tiwari, A., Chan, S., & Law, B. (2002). Stakeholder involvement in curriculum planning: Responding to healthcare reform. *Nurse Educator, 27*(6), 265-270.

Van Ort, S., & Townsend, J. (2002). University community-based nursing education and nursing accreditation by the Commission on Collegiate Nursing Education. *Journal of Professional Nursing, 18*(2), 78-84.

Vilakazi, S., Chabeli, M., & Roos, S. (2000). Integration of the primary health care approach into a community nursing science curriculum. *Curationis, 23*(4), 39-53.

Wenzel, L.S., Briggs, K.L., & Puryear, B.L. (1998). Portfolio: Authentic assessment in the age of the curriculum revolution. *Journal of Nursing Education, 37*(5), 208-212.

Westmoreland, D., & Hays, B.J. (2002). The health systems nurse specialist curriculum: Collaborating across specialties to prepare nurse leaders. *Nursing Education Perspectives, 23*(4), 172–177.

Woodtli, M.A., & Breslin, E.T. (2002).Violence-related content in the nursing curriculum: A follow-up national survey. *Journal of Nursing Education, 41*(8), 340-348.

Yearwood, E., Singleton, J., Feldman, H.R., & Colombraro, G. (2001). A case study in implementing CQI in a nursing education program. *Journal of Professional Nursing, 17*(6), 297-304.

Yurchuck, R., & Brower, H.T. (1994). Faculty preparation for gerontological nursing. *Journal of Gerontological Nursing, 20*(1), 17-24.

Creating an Evidence-based Practice for Nurse Educators

CHAPTER SIX
FUNCTION AS A CHANGE AGENT AND LEADER

Nurse educators function as change agents and leaders when they conceptualize new curriculum models, design innovative educational experiences, and form interprofessional partnerships to create a preferred future for nursing education, the nursing profession, and health care delivery systems. They use their leadership skills to envision new realities for preparing graduates for the ever-changing, complex health care environment in which they will practice.

Nurse educators need to possess the knowledge and skill sets necessary to function effectively in diverse health care and educational environments, and develop collaborative partnerships with practice colleagues to enhance student learning. During a time of unrelenting change in health care and educational systems, as well as critical shortages in nurses and nurse educators, effective leadership is needed from nurse educators. Nurse educators can demonstrate leadership and function as role models in their student relationships (Astin & Astin, 2000), in their relationships with one another and their practice colleagues, and within their institutions. Specifically, to exhibit competence as a change agent and leader, a nurse educator:

- Models cultural sensitivity when advocating for change
- Integrates a long-term, innovative, and creative perspective into the nurse educator role
- Participates in interdisciplinary efforts to address health care and educational needs regionally, nationally, and internationally
- Evaluates organizational effectiveness in nursing education
- Implements strategies for organizational change
- Provides leadership in the parent institution as well as in the nursing program to enhance the visibility of nursing and its contributions to the academic community
- Promotes innovative practices in educational environments
- Develops leadership skills to shape and implement change

Review of the Literature

There were two major themes that emerged from this review of the literature about educators serving as change agents and leaders: 1) leading and managing change in the health care system, and 2) developing an effective leadership style and skills. During the time frame in which this literature review was focused (1992-2004), there were limited research-based articles relevant to the expected competencies of nurse educators as change agents and leaders. Many articles focused on the changing health care system and the need for nurse educators to have knowledge and skill in functioning within the health care system to prepare nursing students to be effective practitioners in the health care arena.

Leading and Managing Change in the Health Care System and the Educational System

Leadership abilities need to be demonstrated by all nurses, including nurse educators, to ensure that nursing advances as a profession and positively impacts health care delivery systems of the future. Themes from the literature relevant to leading and managing the changing health care system included the need for nurse educators to be knowledgeable of the changing health care system, to actively and creatively participate in leadership roles in interprofessional efforts to design new health care systems, and to better prepare graduates to be effective practitioners in these systems.

Brzytwa, Copeland, and Hewson (2000) surveyed nurse educators and employers of new graduates (N = 292) to determine the perceived importance of the practice of nursing competencies (e.g., communicating effectively with clients, engaging clients in self-care), and the business of nursing competencies (e.g., distinguishing between reimbursement mechanisms, needing to select cost-effective diagnostic tests and treatments) in managed care settings. Findings indicated that both employers and nurse educators rated practice of nursing competencies as being most important and most evident in recent nursing graduates, while they rated the business of nursing competencies as less important and most lacking in nursing graduates. These findings lend support to the concern that nurse educators and employers do not find teaching the business of nursing competencies to be as important as practice of nursing competencies even though the literature would suggest that understanding the business of nursing has become increasingly important to effective practice. However, the findings did not give any indication of why educators and employers feel this way. The authors postulated that a fear of change may underlie this reluctance to change teaching practices as educators may not be knowledgeable themselves of the desired business competencies. To practice effectively in the health care system and advocate for their patients, nurses must understand the business side of nursing practice. Nurse educators have a responsibility to be knowledgeable in these business competencies and provide the leadership required to design curricula that introduce students, even at the undergraduate level, to the knowledge and skills required to understand the business of nursing.

The changing practice environment also mandates that health care professionals are able to work in interdisciplinary teams to provide care that is integrated, continuous, and reliable (Institute of Medicine, 2003). Nurse educators must be knowledgeable enough of the practice environment to design new curricula to ensure that graduates have the requisite skills in areas that have been defined by the Institute of Medicine (2003) as essential for health care professionals – patient-centered care, evidence-based practice, quality improvement, interdisciplinary practice, and informatics.

Triolo, Pozehl, and Mahaffey (1997) stated that educators in academic health centers have many opportunities to provide campus leadership within the university environment, as well as influence changes in the health care system. They raised the question, though, of how many faculty actually have the skills required to participate in leading such change efforts. Participating in interdisciplinary task groups, which are commonly found in academic health centers, requires skills in negotiation, conflict resolution, and power-brokering. The higher education environment itself has become an increasingly competitive arena in which educators need the leadership skills required to acquire and maintain scarce resources, and guide the academic restructuring that so many campuses are experiencing. Triolo et al. described the following nine key leadership competencies as essential for nurse educators to provide leadership in these complex environments: "global perspective, superb communication skills, organizational improvement strategies, conflict management, systems thinking, personal mastery, interpersonal mastery, team skills, political savvy" (p. 151). Faculty development strategies to achieve these competencies include: providing opportunities for mentoring; facilitating membership on boards, teams, and task groups; providing feedback, and supporting formal education opportunities. The authors emphasized that the development of faculty leadership competencies must be planned, not left to chance. Educators who are able to display these leadership competencies will be role models for nursing students.

Ciesla and Lovejoy (1997) noted that the following teaching practices are increasingly significant if educators are to prepare graduates to be effective practitioners: inspire the spirit of inquiry and cooperative learning in students; design learning experiences that respect the diverse learning needs of students; develop evaluation strategies to measure effectively student achievement of curriculum competencies; exhibit vision and innovation in designing learning experiences; exhibit enthusiasm and accomplishment in the educator role, and be supportive of students. Booth (1994) stated that nurse educators need to exhibit the characteristics of a leader, motivator, master teacher, and expert role model.

Porter-O'Grady and Malloch (2003) described the current changes in the health care system as chaotic, complex, and multidirectional, and asserted that new models of leadership are required. They stated that leaders in this chaotic environment need to understand the complexity of change and that change will be evident on a daily basis.

In this time of accelerated, nonlinear change in the health care system, nurse leaders, including educators, need leadership competencies that can transform health care organizations and educational programs.

Menix (2000) conducted a critical review of nursing, business, and higher education literature on the management of change. Results suggested that planned change was emphasized in all three disciplines' educational literature, but that there was limited information emphasizing nonlinear change. While seven years have elapsed since this article was published, the findings still point to the importance of educators reviewing and revising current curricula to reflect more focus on nonlinear change in complex, adaptive systems.

Grossman and Valiga (2005) indicated that nursing leadership for reshaping future health care systems and improving client care will require personal leadership qualities as well as organizational leadership qualities. Nurse educators must be committed to continuing to develop their own leadership abilities, as well as mentoring students in leadership development. Being politically aware, actively involved in leadership roles in professional organizations, and displaying advocacy skills are some examples by which nurse educators can model leadership behaviors for students.

The multicultural world in which we now live requires nurses to deliver culturally focused health care and to be sensitive to cultural implications when advocating for change. Ryan, Carlton, and Ali (2000) conducted a descriptive survey to examine curricular trends in transcultural nursing in baccalaureate and graduate nursing programs in the United States. Study results indicated that transcultural nursing concepts have been integrated in most nursing courses, but that there is variation as to the content and depth of the material. The authors recommended that nurse educators develop competency in transcultural nursing to function as leaders and role models for nursing students.

Developing Effective Leadership Styles and Skills

Several research studies focused on identifying the most effective leadership styles or skills for educators and deans. For example, Shieh, Mills, and Waltz (2001) investigated the influence of nursing deans' and nursing directors' transformational and transactional leadership styles on nursing faculty job satisfaction in baccalaureate and associate degree nursing programs in Taiwan in a cross-sectional survey that was mailed to a convenience sample of nursing faculty ($N = 233$). The faculty completed two survey tools, the Multifactor Leadership Questionnaire and the Nursing Faculty Satisfaction Questionnaire. Both instruments were translated into Chinese, and content validity and reliability were established for the translated instruments. Cronbach's alpha for the scales and subscales ranged from .71 to .94. Findings indicated that dean and director leadership styles that utilized 1) idealized influence, producing trust and clarity of goals; 2) intellectual stimulation, providing focus on problem-solving solutions; and 3) contingent rewards for faculty, based upon performance, significantly (idealized influence and contigent reward, $p < .001$; intellectual stimulation, $p < .05$) and positively predicted faculty job satisfaction and satisfaction with leadership. Based upon these findings, the authors stated that a leadership training program that highlights idealized influence, intellectual stimulation, and contingent reward styles of leadership should be offered to prepare effective leaders in nursing education.

According to the literature, gender differences among leaders may also affect faculty perceptions of effective leadership styles. Rosser (2003) examined faculty and staff members' perceptions of effective leadership that may explain the way men and women lead academic units in higher education settings. Faculty and staff ($N = 865$) were asked to evaluate the performance of their deans in relation to leadership abilities. Results suggested that faculty and staff perceive that men and women did differ in their leadership patterns. Women were more likely to be perceived to enhance the quality of education in their unit; engage in research; participate in community, and professional projects; encourage institutional diversity; and effectively manage staff and resources. Female deans were rated as more effective leaders than male deans in every dimension of leadership.

The perceived leadership styles of educators can also influence student perceptions of instructor effectiveness and student engagement. In a study outside the discipline of nursing, the transformational leadership style of instructors was examined by Harvey, Royal, and

Stout (2003). A convenience sample of 120 undergraduate students rated their instructors' performance in the following categories: charisma, intellectual stimulation, and individual consideration. Intellectual stimulation and charisma explained 66.3% of the variance in the performance of the instructors as perceived by the students. Intellectual stimulation and individual consideration predicted 55.1% of the variance in student involvement.

Effective leadership abilities need to be exhibited by all nurses for nursing to advance as a profession and impact further development of the health delivery system (Grossman & Valiga, 2005). Nurse educators have responsibility for designing programs and curricula that ensure students are exposed to relevant leadership content so they can develop the required skills. In a descriptive study, Lemire (2001) validated the knowledge and skills needed by effective leaders in a sample of 500 nursing administrators, educators, and students. Visionary, achiever, critical thinker, communicator, and mentor were identified as the major characteristics of an effective leader, especially during a time of major change and turmoil in the health care system.

While the characteristics identified by Lemire (2001) for leaders are important, it is likely that leaders of the future will need to possess additional competencies. In a qualitative study, Starck, Warner, and Kotarba (1999) interviewed six deans at top ranking nursing graduate programs in the United States to identify skills required for academic leadership in the twenty-first century. Current leadership skills identified by these leaders in academia included functioning as a director of a centralized structure, proactively responding to problems, and sharing information with faculty to negotiate good decision-making. The deans identified that future leadership skills will require being a consensus builder, a risk-taker, and an interactive empowerer of faculty. Their collective vision for twenty-first century nurse educators included being more entrepreneurial, engaging in more educational outreach, being expert in the use of technology, and developing a more business-like accountability in their approach to nursing education.

Hartman (2000) examined the leadership behaviors in a sample of 46 men and women in senior management positions. The personality factor of warmth was a robust and consistent predictor of leadership effectiveness. Warmth was significantly tied to overall leadership and people high on warmth were described as easygoing, adaptable, warmhearted, cooperative, frank, attentive to people, expressive, trustful, and participating. Data also supported that warmth is a necessary but not a sufficient condition for effective leadership.

Emotional intelligence is thought to be a major contributing factor to effective leadership in part by helping individuals to become more collaborative team members (Goleman, 1998). Vitello-Cicciu (2003) examined the concept of emotional intelligence and leadership behaviors of 50 nurse leaders. The nurse leaders who had higher emotional intelligence scores reported reading self-help books, practicing meditation, avoiding taking things personally, and managing stress. They also appeared to have more self-awareness about both their own emotions and others'. Effective leadership behaviors, grounded in emotional intelligence, are needed to develop and foster the high-energy teams needed in today's changing health care system.

Identified Gaps in the Literature

The review of the literature demonstrated the importance of nurse educators functioning as change agents and leaders in the health care system and higher education arena. The rapidly changing health care delivery system requires educators to take a leadership role in designing educational experiences that prepare graduates for practice in new and complex health care systems. In order to assume this leadership role as a change agent, nurse educators need to develop a knowledge base of health care systems and the business of nursing, so that they can effectively develop experiences that facilitate students learning how to function in complex health care delivery systems.

As there is little evidence-based literature on developing the change agent and leadership competencies of nurse educators in the higher education environment, further research is needed to develop and validate best practices for this competency. The rapid changes occurring in education and health care delivery are taking place in an information-driven, global society. Nurse educators need to be able to function in a culturally diverse world, as well as exhibit competence in the use of information technology, so that they can emerge as leaders in health care and education.

Priorities for Future Research

The following questions are offered to stimulate research that will enhance our understanding of the nurse educator competency of functioning as a change agent and leader:

- What are the best practices for helping nurse educators attain the skills necessary to function as change agents and leaders in the nursing profession?

- What are the most effective mentoring approaches for developing future leaders in nursing education?

- How can educators most effectively teach students about the concepts of systems thinking, complexity, outcomes measurement, quality improvement, information management, and the business of nursing?

- What are the essential skills, attitudes, and knowledge for nurse educators to be able to model cultural sensitivity when advocating for change?

References

Astin, W., & Astin, H. (2002). Introduction to *Leadership reconsidered: Engaging higher education in social change.* Battle Creek, MI: W. K. Kellogg Foundation.

Booth, R. (1994). A mandate for nursing education leadership change. *Journal of Professional Nursing, 10*(6), 335-341.

Brzytwa, E., Copeland, L., & Hewson, M. (2000). Managed care education: A needs assessment of employers and educators of nurses. *Journal of Nursing Education, 39*(5), 197-205.

Ciesla, S., & Lovejoy, C. (1997). Peer review: A method for developing faculty leaders. *Nurse Educator, 22*(6), 41-47.

Goleman, P. (1998). *Working with emotional intelligence.* New York: Bantam Books.

Grossman, S., & Valiga, T.M. (2005). *The new leadership challenge: Creating the future of nursing (2nd ed.).* Philadelphia: F.A. Davis Company.

Hartman, L. (2000). A psychological analysis of leadership effectiveness. *Strategy and Leadership, 27*(6), 30-32.

Harvey, S., Royal, M., & Stout, D. (2003). Instructor's transformational leadership: University student attitudes and ratings. *Psychological Reports, 92*(2), 395-396.

Insitute of Medicine. (2003). *Health professions education: A bridge to quality.* Washington, DC: National Academies Press.

Lemire, J. A. (2001). Preparing nurse leaders: A leadership education model. *Nursing Leadership Forum, 6*(2), 39-44.

Menix, K. (2000). Educating to manage the accelerated change environment effectively: Part 1. *Journal for Nurses in Staff Development, 16*(6), 282-288.

Porter-O'Grady, T. & Malloch, K. (2003). *Quantum leadership: A textbook of new leadership.* Boston: Jones and Bartlett Publishers.

Rosser, V. (2003). Faculty and staff members' perceptions of effective leadership: Are there differences between women and men leaders? *Equity and Excellence in Education, 36*(1), 71-81.

Ryan, M., Carlton, K., & Ali, N. (2000). Transcultural nursing concepts and experiences in nursing curricula. *Journal of Transcultural Nursing, 11*(4), 300-307.

Shieh, H., Mills, M., & Waltz, C. (2001). Academic leadership style predictors for nursing faculty job satisfaction in Taiwan. *Journal of Nursing Education, 40*(5), 203-209.

Starck, P., Warner, A. & Kotarba, J. (1999). 21st leadership in nursing education: The need for trifocals. *Journal of Professional Nursing, 15*(5), 265-269.

Triolo, P., Pozehl, B., & Mahaffey, T. (1997). Development of leadership within the university and beyond: Challenges to faculty and their development. *Journal of Professional Nursing, 13,* (3), 149-153.

Vitello-Cicciu, J. (2003). Innovative leadership through emotional intelligence. *Journal of Nursing Management, 34*(10), 28-32.

Creating an Evidence-based Practice for Nurse Educators

CHAPTER SEVEN

PURSUE CONTINUOUS QUALITY IMPROVEMENT IN THE NURSE EDUCATOR ROLE

The current nursing education environment is marked by changing student demographics, a market driven by economics, an explosion of technology, and complex care delivery in multiple health care environments (Lindemann, 2000). An increasing shortage of experienced nurse educators threatens to impact the quality of our educational programs and limits the number of students who can be accepted into programs at a time when the demand for nurses continues to rise (Kelly, 2002). There needs to be a sufficient number of nurse educators who are academically prepared to teach in classroom and clinical settings, engage in research and scholarly activities, and provide service to the institution and the profession. Furthermore, to maintain effectiveness as educators, faculty need to keep current in clinical practice, teaching and learning strategies, technology advancements, and educational and societal issues that impact the practice of nursing and nursing education.

Nurse educators recognize that their role is multidimensional and successful implementation of the educator role requires a commitment to developing and maintaining the competence inherent to the role. New nurse educators, who typically have strong clinical backgrounds, can benefit from mentoring by experienced educators as they assume the educator role. In addition, experienced educators need support from professional colleagues to meet their own development needs.

The National League for Nursing's position statement on *Lifelong Learning for Nursing Faculty* encourages all educators to participate in ongoing development activities connected to their educator role (NLN, 2001). Nurse educators must value lifelong learning and acknowledge that, as they evolve from novices to experts in their role as educators, professional development needs will vary. To effectively pursue continuous quality improvement in the educator role, the nurse educator:

- Demonstrates a commitment to lifelong learning
- Recognizes that career enhancement needs and activities change as experience is gained in the role
- Participates in professional development opportunities that increase one's effectiveness in the role
- Balances the teaching, scholarship, and service demands inherent in the role of the educator and member of an academic institution
- Uses feedback gained from self, peer, student, and administrative evaluation to improve role effectiveness
- Engages in activities that promote one's socialization to the role
- Uses knowledge of legal and ethical issues relevant to higher education and nursing education as a basis for influencing, designing, and implementing policies and procedures related to students, faculty, and the educational environment
- Mentors and supports faculty colleagues

Review of the Literature

A review of the literature on continuous quality improvement in the nurse educator role revealed that little attention has been given to this topic and only a handful of research studies have been conducted on it. However, the literature does cluster around several themes that enhance our understanding of lifelong professional development of nurse educators: 1) role strain in nurse educators; 2) developmental needs of novice educators; 3) developmental needs of experienced educators; 4) faculty development strategies; 5) evaluation of educator effectiveness; and 6) socialization into the role of educator.

Role Strain in Nurse Educators

Nurse educators practice in the dynamic, ever-changing environments of health care and education. The competing, multiple demands present in these environments can lead to role strain. An understanding of role demands and stressors can help educators better cope with the challenges of the role. Magnussen (1997) stated that the expectations of teaching, scholarship, and service, in addition to maintaining clinical competence, can cause nurse educators to feel overwhelmed. She recommended that educators design and implement a career plan to facilitate professional development and increase the likelihood of success in meeting role expectations. Others have suggested that orientation programs that identify role expectations and resources can be helpful to both novice and experienced faculty alike in decreasing potential role strain (Boyden, 2000; Morin & Ashton, 1998).

One of the demands of the educator role is maintaining clinical relevancy. However, there has been limited research into the stressors related specifically to the role of clinical nursing faculty. Oermann (1998), identifying the need to study the work-related stress associated with the role of clinical faculty, conducted a descriptive, exploratory design study to identify the most common stressors. A total of 226 undergraduate clinical nursing faculty from programs located in the midwestern United States completed an instrument designed to measure work-related stressors. Content validity and reliability of the instrument was established and found to be acceptable. The most commonly identified stressors for clinical faculty included meeting the job expectations of their clinical teaching role, coping with the physical and emotional demands of the role, having the demands of the role interfere with personally important activities, finding the time to maintain clinical competence, and teaching students who are ill-prepared for the clinical experience. Clinical faculty from baccalaureate programs reported higher levels of role stress than did clinical faculty from associate degree programs in the areas of workload, job expectations, and interference with personally important activities. To help decrease role stress and strain, Oermann recommended that clinical faculty be mentored to help them understand and cope with the responsibilities and demands of clinical teaching, and that administrators identify ways to recognize clinical teaching excellence.

The potential for role strain is evident in nurse educators in other countries as well. In a descriptive, correlational study based upon Kanter's theory of organizational empowerment, Sarmiento, Laschinger, and Iwasiw (2004) explored the relationship between faculty satisfaction, burnout, and empowerment among Canadian college nurse educators (N = 89). In this population, job satisfaction was positively affected by low levels of emotional exhaustion (an element of burnout) and high levels of empowerment ($p = 0.0001$). Overall, these educators reported feeling moderately empowered in their role. The authors suggested that strategies that increase educators' empowerment in their role, such as access to resources and information, would lead to greater job satisfaction.

Cahill (1997) addressed the increasing complexity of the nurse teacher role in the United Kingdom as a result of nursing education moving into the higher education system. In a qualitative study focused on identifying factors related to teacher workload, Cahill conducted focus group interviews of key stakeholders in the educational system, including teachers, students, college administrators, and regulatory commissioners. The results of this preliminary study clearly indicated that there are competing demands on the nurse teachers' role – to provide quality educational experiences for students, be clinically competent, and contribute to higher education's research mission. As the nurse teacher role continues to evolve in the United Kingdom, further study is required to understand the tensions that exist among these competing demands and the effect that these varied expectations will have on the skill set required by nurse teachers in this new educational environment.

Despite the role strain and workload issues that have been identified for nurse educators, many educators find the role to be professionally and personally rewarding. Additional research into how to effectively reduce role strain and address the developmental needs of educators is warranted, so as to enhance recruitment and retention of qualified educators.

Developmental Needs of the Novice Educator

Characteristics of effective educators have been identified by many authors, including Choudhry (1992), Dienemann and Shaffer (1992), and Fairbrother (1996). These authors reported on studies conducted to determine the characteristics that are indicative of quality teachers. These characteristics include: 1) being committed to teaching and intellectual inquiry; 2) demonstrating knowledge and love of the subject; 3) enjoying interactions with students; 4) being available to students; 5) being conscientious when evaluating students' work; 6) demonstrating fairness; 7) exhibiting professional competence; 8) being well prepared; 9) using innovative teaching practices; and 10) role modeling excellent communication skills.

The novice nurse educator may find developing the characteristics of an effective teacher to be overwhelming while teaching a full-time load, advising students, staying professionally current, participating in scholarly activities, and providing service to the institution and the profession. Mentoring can help the novice educator achieve balance among these multiple demands (Adams, 2002).

The experiences of novice educators, however, may not necessarily include a mentoring relationship. Siler and Kleiner (2001) conducted a phenomenological study about the experiences of educators in their first year of full-time employment within an institution. A common theme that emerged from the study was that of expectations. These expectations may be the educators' own expectations of their new role or the expectations of students and faculty.

In Siler and Kleiner's study (2001), there were a total of 12 participants, six of whom were novice educators and six of whom were experienced. They were employed in 11 different institutions. In this particular article, Siler and Kleiner chose to report the perspective of the novice educators. Hermeneutic analysis indicated that the novice educators found themselves in an unfamiliar role in an unfamiliar academic environment. The workload was greater than anticipated, they struggled to find answers to their teaching questions, and all experienced concerns about their performance. They expected to receive guidance from their more experienced colleagues, but found that even experienced faculty, while caring, had difficulty articulating how to teach effectively. Mentors were assigned to each novice educator, but the relationships did not develop for a number of reasons (e.g., scheduling conflicts, personality differences). None of the novice educators received a formal peer evaluation the first year of their teaching; rather, their primary source of feedback was from students. The authors concluded that the lack of dialogue that exists about the teaching role contributes to a sense of isolation and that there is a need for formal academic preparation for nurse educators.

Kavoosi, Elman, and Mauch (1995) conducted a descriptive, correlational study to identify the extent to which senior faculty engaged in mentoring of junior faculty and the level of administrative support provided for mentoring activities. A total of 389 MSN nursing faculty and 80 administrators in NLNAC-accredited programs completed two surveys – the faculty completed the Alleman Mentoring Scales Questionnaire and the administrators completed the Administrative Data Questionnaire. The majority of the faculty (75%) respondents reported mentoring junior faculty in their work environment and that they were most likely to engage in mentoring activities that "taught" the job, demonstrated trust, or sponsored the junior faculty for professional opportunities. There was no statistically significant relationship identified between faculty mentoring activities and administrative support. It appeared that the majority of mentoring being reported by senior faculty was informal and not necessarily influenced by any formal expectation of administration. Despite the lack of correlation between administrative support and mentoring activities, administrators were encouraged to develop a work environment that expects and rewards mentoring activities. Limitations of this study included only getting the mentors' perspective on their mentoring activities and the potential for different interpretations of the definition of mentoring among respondents.

Although the educator role can seem stressful and overwhelming, novice faculty have also reported positive aspects of practicing in the nursing education environment. Clifford's (1995) exploratory study about the role of the nurse teacher in the United Kingdom revealed that nurse teachers were most positive about "learner contact, seeing learners develop skills, influencing practice, the challenge of change, and autonomy" (p. 13).

The preparation of novice educators to function in the faculty role has also been investigated. Davis, Dearman, Schwab, and Kitchens (1992) conducted a study to determine novice educators' (N = 427) perceptions of the competencies needed for the role, to what extent the competencies were exhibited by the novice educators, and how novice educators developed the competencies. Novice educators were defined as those with no more than two years' experience in the role. Study participants completed demographic data and the Nurse Faculty Competency Questionnaire, which is an instrument that contains 43 competency statements about the faculty role. Content validity of the instrument was established, but the reliability of the instrument was not addressed. Findings indicated that many of the novice educators agreed with the competencies associated with the teaching function of the role, but did not agree with the competencies related to the research and service functions of the role. The novice educators were most comfortable with demonstrating the clinical aspects of the teaching role. The authors' indicated that this particular population of educators did not appear to be educationally prepared for the role, with 23% prepared at the baccalaureate level. Of those who had a master's or doctoral degree, only two thirds had any formal academic courses to prepare them for the role. They concluded there is a need to socialize graduate students into the tripartite role (teaching, research, and service) of faculty.

Choudhry (1992) also investigated novice educator competencies among faculty (N = 268) from community college and university nursing programs located in Ontario. The researcher-developed Likert-type instrument contained 96 competencies developed from the literature. Face validity was established and a Cronbach's alpha of greater than .88 was reported for all subscales. There were significant differences in the competencies based upon type of institution, with faculty in the community colleges rating student evaluation, facilitating clinical experiences, and acting as an adviser higher than university faculty. University faculty rated research competencies higher than faculty in community colleges rated research. Similar to Davies et al. (1992), Choudhry concluded that novice educators require academic preparation for the role and socialization to the role.

Nugent, Bradshaw, and Kito (1999) conducted a study to determine what factors influenced novice educators' perception of self-efficacy in the teaching role. They defined novice educators to be those who had five or less years of teaching experience. A total of 346 novice baccalaureate nursing faculty from NLNAC-accredited programs participated in the study, completing the Self-Efficacy Toward Teaching Inventory (SETTI) as adapted by the researchers for this study. Internal consistency of the revised version of the instrument was reported to be a .95 alpha coefficient. This particular population of educators reported feeling confident in their ability to teach, possibly because the majority of them had three or more years of teaching experience and reported receiving formal academic preparation for the role. The findings of this study indicated that the self-efficacy of novice educators can be positively affected by academic preparation and teaching experience. Limitations of the study included reliance on self-reported data and sample size. In addition to formal preparation for the educator role, the authors also recommended mentoring by experienced faculty.

Because of the complexity of the faculty role, Magnussen (1997) recommended that all new faculty have a professional development plan that projects an academic career trajectory. She sets out a five-year career development plan that new faculty can use as a guide and recommends the implementation of a mentoring program. In addition to teaching and research expectations, novice faculty also need to know about the expectations of committee and faculty governance responsibilities, as well as community and recruitment events that may occur on weekends or in the evening (Adams, 2002). Novice faculty also need to understand how these various aspects of the faculty role – teaching, research, and service – will be evaluated in the promotion and tenure process (Riner & Billings, 1999), so that they can construct a faculty development plan that will help ensure their institutional success in achieving promotion and tenure.

Developmental Needs of the Experienced Educator

While the developmental needs of novice educators have received some attention in the literature, the developmental needs of experienced educators have been less researched. Experienced faculty do have developmental needs, especially when they enter a new academic environment or strive to meet the requirements for successfully navigating the tenure and promotion system. Because of the lack of literature on the needs of experienced faculty, especially those teaching primarily in graduate programs, Morin & Ashton (1998) conducted a study to determine the characteristics of orientation programs for this group and which aspects of the orientation program were most helpful to faculty as they transitioned into a new academic position. Most faculty (79%) reported receiving an orientation and rated information about the educational environment (e.g., curriculum and student advisement), faculty role, social milieu, and support systems as most helpful. The authors surmised that orientation programs can increase faculty productivity and decrease role strain. They recommended additional research to identify the most effective length of time for orientation programs and the level of comprehensiveness most likely to meet faculty needs.

Faculty Development Strategies

Faculty development strategies are essential for developing competent educators. Novice faculty who need development regarding teaching skills, mid-career faculty who want to expand their pedagogical literacy, and expert faculty who wish to develop as leaders need to stay abreast of what is current in nursing education (Lane, 1996). It is common for nursing academic units to have funds allocated for faculty development, although such funds may be limited. These funds are intended for faculty use to maintain knowledge and competence in their clinical specialty, as well as develop their competence as nurse educators. Funds are usually divided among faculty members with full-time faculty members receiving greater support than part-time or adjunct faculty. Many institutions are not able to provide development funds for part-time and adjunct faculty. With resources being limited, it is important that administrators consider a variety of strategies to facilitate faculty development.

Faculty development can occur in a number of ways. For example, on-campus workshops or seminars, courses in advanced degree programs, online and audio/web modules, peer support systems, mentoring programs, sabbaticals, and the use of campus and academic unit resource centers where faculty can find necessary support are strategies that can be used to promote faculty development (Lane, 1996). Collaborative faculty research teams, writing groups, and journal clubs are examples of how faculty research development needs can be met (Magnussen, 1997). Smolen (1996) supported faculty development, but cautioned that "work load, insufficient institutional financing, ... faculty scheduling, and lack of release time" (p. 92) may prevent faculty from participating in development activities.

The areas for faculty development are numerous. Boyden (2000) identified several challenges that are currently facing nursing education and require continuous quality improvement on the part of educators: changing student demographics; increasing use of technology in education; decreasing resources, and increasing emphasis on quality undergraduate education. Faculty also need continued development in international and interdisciplinary educational efforts (Adams, 2002). Evidence-based practice and clinical information systems are other examples of practice demands that require continued faculty development.

Staff nurses are now using personal digital assistants (PDAs) to input patient care notes and vital signs, and carrying cell phones on the clinical unit to facilitate communication and the management of patient care. Within the university, a classroom teacher may see "... teleconferencing, electronic mail, multimedia applications, distance learning" (Boyden, 2000, p. 106). It is also important to remember that part-time and adjunct faculty are as much in need of development as full-time faculty.

Evaluation of Educator Effectiveness

Evaluating educator effectiveness with the goal of improving performance in the role was a major theme in the literature. The educator role is multidimensional; to effectively evaluate performance in it requires consideration of all the domains and dimensions of the role.

Dienemann and Shaffer (1992) conducted a study of the policies, procedures, and performance appraisal forms of schools of nursing that had graduate programs (N = 86) to identify the domains, dimensions, and subdimensions used for measurement in educator performance appraisals in academia and to identify the elements of an effective performance appraisal system. The traditionally identified domains of teaching, research, and service were supported by content analysis of the data. The most common dimensions of the teaching domain were teaching in the classroom, clinical teaching, and student advising. The most frequently identified dimensions of research were publications, oral presentations, grant writing, and conducting research. The most frequently identified dimensions of the service domain were service to the profession, community, school of nursing, and university. While subdimensions for each domain were reported by some of the schools, these varied and had less agreement among the programs. Dienemann and Shaffer concluded that expectations of the educator role varied amongst nursing programs and were dependent upon the environment within which the educator was employed. Expectations also varied depending upon the educator's career stage. They noted that the majority of the performance appraisal forms reviewed were summative in nature and urged the development of formative evaluation systems that could be used to guide junior faculty in the promotion and tenure process.

The evaluation of educator effectiveness is conducted in numerous ways. It is important that the educator understand who will be evaluating her or his performance (Ward-Griffin & Brown, 1992). The literature addressed self-evaluation, peer evaluation, student evaluation, and administrative evaluation.

Self-Evaluation. One method of evaluation that was mentioned frequently in the literature was self-evaluation through reflection on one's practice as a teacher. Research studies about reflective practice and its effectiveness in helping educators develop their teaching skills were minimal. Some of the literature offered educators tools to use in documenting their effectiveness as teachers, such as teaching portfolios (Oermann, 1999).

Burnard (1995) conducted a qualitative study with 12 nurse educators, interviewing them about the use of reflective practice in teaching. The respondents appeared to focus their responses more on the use of reflective practice in their roles as clinicians than in their roles as educators. While most of the nurse educators professed to seeing some value to reflecting on their practice as teachers, as well as value in teaching reflection to students, many indicated that they did not have a clear understanding on how to model reflective practice for their students. Burnard recommended additional research to add to the minimal empirical evidence reported in the literature to help educators use reflective practice in a meaningful and effective manner.

Peer Evaluation. Evaluation by one's peers is frequently cited as a means by which educators can gain information to help them develop in the teaching role. The effectiveness of peer evaluation, however, was seldom addressed in the literature during the time frame covered by this review.

Crawford (1998) conducted a study among NLNAC-accredited baccalaureate nursing schools to assess the use of peer evaluation of classroom teaching, determine faculty perceptions about the value of peer review in the classroom, and identify the behaviors that faculty thought could be evaluated through classroom observation of teaching. Respondents indicated that peer evaluation in the classroom setting could be a valuable means of assessing faculty teaching performance, and they cited the following behaviors as those most likely to be appropriate to observe in a classroom review process: content knowledge, organizational abilities and clarity of presentation, demonstration of respect for students, enthusiasm, and communication abilities. Crawford made the following recommendations for further discussion: clarification of the purpose for observation of faculty in the classroom, as faculty and administrators appear to have different perceptions of the purpose; number of observations that would be most appropriate for evaluation of teaching effectiveness; appropriate weighting of classroom observations to measure teaching effectiveness in relation to other means of evaluation; and further research on tool effectiveness for faculty evaluation.

Johnston (1996) proposed that an educator's ability to function effectively in a group is an important skill. She then developed a tool that can be used to evaluate an educator's effectiveness as a group member who deserves to be valued and rewarded. Face and content validity of this peer evaluation tool was established and it was pilot tested with a group of faculty. While the author stated that the feedback received was used to edit the tool, further details of the outcome of the pilot test were not provided.

Student Evaluation. Student evaluations of educator performance in the classroom and clinical settings are frequently used as one, and at times the only, means of determining the educator's effectiveness in the teaching role. There is little in the research literature, however, that focuses on the use of reliable and valid tools by which student evaluations are conducted. Reeve (1994) developed an instrument that undergraduate students could use to evaluate clinical instructors, pilot testing the instrument to determine reliability and validity. She cautioned that when reviewing the results of clinical evaluations, it is important to keep in mind that most clinical groups are small (consisting of 10 or fewer students), and that one overwhelmingly positive or negative rater can skew the results. There were no research studies found in the literature that addressed the topic of the reliability and validity of tools used for student evaluation of classroom teaching.

Administrative Evaluation. Research literature on the evaluation of nurse educators by administrators is very limited; in fact, only one study that addressed this topic was found. In a study about evaluating faculty through the use of classroom observation, Crawford (1998) surveyed school of nursing administrators as well as nursing faculty to determine how classroom observation was used in the evaluation process for faculty review and promotion. Only 54% of the administrators surveyed used the classroom observations to provide feedback to faculty for development purposes. In 65% of the schools that conducted reviews in the classroom, administrators were observers. Some administrators indicated that faculty viewed the review process as "threatening" and questioned the value of what was primarily a subjective process. Administrators suggested that having guidelines for conducting observations in the classroom would be one way of making the review process more consistent and meaningful.

Socialization into the Role of Educator

Expert nurses entering the clinical or classroom teaching environment for the first time may suddenly find themselves feeling like they are novices (Lindemann, 2000). Because of this, the literature strongly supports a mentoring environment (Boyden, 2000; Davis et al., 1992; DeNeff, 2002; Johnson, 2002; Kelly, 2002; Lindemann, 2000; Magnussen, 1997; Mundt, 2001; Riner & Billings, 1999; Smolen, 1996) to help the individual adjust to the new role.

Clinical Teaching. During the last 15 to 20 years, many graduate programs decreased or eliminated their educational preparation of nurse educators in favor of preparing nurses with advanced clinical practice skills (Hermann, 1997). There has been an assumption in the discipline that expert clinicians make excellent clinical teachers. However, there are issues of role strain compounded by a lack of understanding of the responsibilities of the educator role, especially when the individual lacks the educational preparation to assume the teaching role (Boyden, 2000; Riner & Billings, 1999). Educators need to know that teaching demands a considerable amount of time and energy; thus, they need to be "teacher ready" (Adams, 2002, p. 3) when they take on this responsibility.

The literature abounds with descriptions of the functions and characteristics of clinical nurse instructors, but there is little in the literature that discusses preparation or role socialization for the clinical instructor. Davies, White, Riley, and Twinn (1996) interviewed students, practitioners, and nurse educators to determine the role functions of clinical nurse teachers. These researchers learned that clinical nurse educators are expected to function as liaisons between the academic setting and the clinical facility, resolve problems with students or staff, provide support to the students and staff, monitor students' progress, inform the staff of student learning needs, negotiate for clinical placements, contribute to the evaluation of the students, and mentor the staff who are helping the students. Many new clinical faculty do not realize that these functions are expectations of the role. Duffy and Watson (2001) conducted an interpretive study on the role of the clinical educator in Scotland. Eighteen nurse teachers participated in the study. The main themes related to the role of nurse teacher in the practice setting that emerged from this study were being a regulator, interpreter, networker, adviser, and supporter.

Ludwick, Dieckman, Herdtner, Dugan, and Roche (1998) stated that clinical teaching can be draining, demanding, and demeaning. Other authors have stated that maintaining clinical expertise and participating in clinical teaching are very time consuming and rarely rewarded, not to mention physically and emotionally draining (Choudhry, 1992; Oermann, 1998). Because there is little interacting with other faculty while teaching in the clinical setting, clinical faculty often feel as if they are teaching in isolation. They may be worried about patient safety issues or they may believe they have access to limited resources to assist them with their teaching role while on the unit.

Smolen (1996) stated that all faculty, but clinical faculty in particular, need support initially as they obtain the necessary experience to fulfill the role. This can be accomplished with a mentoring program and a competency-based orientation program that includes specific goals and objectives (Vezina et al., 1996). In the mentoring program, new clinical faculty should be allowed to observe experienced clinical faculty as they teach students, and there should be an experienced faculty in the facility at all times who can serve as a resource person to the new faculty as needed.

Classroom Teaching. New classroom faculty have many issues with which they must cope, especially if their graduate education did not prepare them for a teaching role. This may be the first time they are exposed to teaching individuals with diverse learning needs, while simultaneously learning about the teaching, scholarship, and service expectations of the role, the amount of time it takes to prepare for a class, and how to keep up with the amount of knowledge required to stay current in education and in one's area of specialty (Love, 1996). Socialization into the faculty role also may include such activities as presenting at conferences, writing grants, conducting research, advising students, and serving on committees. New faculty may benefit from finding a mentor to help them understand and manage all the demands of the faculty role. In socializing new faculty to the role, the mentor can help the faculty understand the amount of time they can expect to allocate to class preparation, especially the first time they are teaching a course. New faculty also need to be socialized into the scholarship role that involves conducting research, writing, publishing, and presenting as well as the service role that includes department and university committee activities (Kotecki & Eddy, 1994; McElroy, 1997).

Identified Gaps in the Literature

The nursing profession is facing a significant shortage of nurse educators. How to effectively prepare future educators and assist them in their professional development are critical issues that must be addressed. This review of the literature revealed several gaps in the research literature related to continuous quality improvement in the educator role.

Overall, there was little research on developing educator competencies, especially as the educator moves along the career trajectory from novice to expert. Furthermore, since the environment in which an educator is employed will impact the competencies that he/she is expected to exhibit, the concept of institutional "fit" and how to achieve it to ensure success and satisfaction in the educator role needs to be studied. Role development needs of adjunct, part-time, and clinical faculty also need to be addressed, especially as the use of part-time and adjunct faculty continues to increase. Finally, formal academic preparation for the nurse educator role was not addressed.

Other areas that lacked attention in the literature were evidence-based practices of the effective evaluation of educators, research on the effectiveness of faculty development and orientation programs, and studies about how to effectively socialize educators to the educational environment and their responsibilities in the academy. It was acknowledged in the literature that role strain was common among nurse educators, thus further discussion about the etiology of stressors and how these stressors differ between novice and experienced educators, as well as how to cope with them, is warranted.

Priorities for Future Research

The following priorities for future research of the educator competency, pursuing continuous quality improvement in the nurse educator role, are recommended:

- What are the most effective curriculum designs for graduate nursing programs and continuing education programs for the purpose of preparing nurse educators?
- In what ways are the competencies of novice nurse educators similar to and different from the competencies of experienced educators?
- What are the professional development needs of adjunct, part-time, and clinical nurse educators in the role of educator?
- How are educator competencies similar and how are they different depending on the type of institutional setting (e.g., research, liberal arts, comprehensive, community college, clinical) and educational program (e.g., doctoral, master's, baccalaureate, associate, vocational, diploma, clinical)?

- What methods most effectively support and guide continued growth and development in the nurse educator role?

- What stressors and coping mechanisms are most significant for nurse educators?

- What methods are most effective for socializing nurses into the role of educator?

- What strategies facilitate initial role socialization and ongoing role development of new faculty with limited knowledge of the academic environment?

- What are the differences in mentoring needed by novice and experienced educators?

References

Adams, K. (2002). *What colleges and universities want in new faculty.* Washington, DC: American Association of Colleges & Universities.

Boyden, K. (2000). Development of new faculty in higher education. *Journal of Professional Nursing, 16*(2), 104-111.

Burnard, P. (1995). Nurse educators' perceptions of reflection and reflective practice: A report of a descriptive study. *Journal of Advanced Nursing, 21*(6), 1167-1174.

Cahill, H. (1997). What should nurse teachers be doing? A preliminary study. *Journal of Advanced Nursing, 26*(1), 146-153.

Choudhry, U. (1992). New nursing faculty: Core competencies for role development. *Journal of Nursing Education, 31*(6), 265-272.

Clifford, C. (1995). The role of nurse teachers: Concerns, conflicts, and challenges. *Nurse Education Today, 15*(1), 11-16.

Crawford, L.H. (1998). Evaluation of nursing faculty through observation. *Journal of Nursing Education, 37*(7), 289-294.

Davies, S., White, E., Riley, E., & Twinn, S. (1996). How can nurse teachers be more effective in practice settings? *Nurse Education Today, 16*(1), 19-27.

Davis, D., Dearman, C., Schwab, C., & Kitchens, E. (1992). Competencies of novice nurse educators. *Journal of Nursing Education, 31*(4), 159-164.

DeNeff, A. (2002). *The Preparing Future Faculty Program: What difference does it make?* Washington, DC: American Association of Colleges & Universities.

Dienemann, J. & Shaffer, C. (1992). Faculty performance appraisal systems: Procedures and criteria. *Journal of Professional Nursing, 8*(3), 148-154.

Duffy, K., & Watson, H. (2001). An interpretive study of the nurse teacher's role in practice placement areas. *Nurse Education Today, 21*(7), 551-558.

Fairbrother, P. (1996). Recognition and assessment of teaching quality. *Nurse Education Today, 16*(1), 69-74.

Hermann, M. (1997). The relationship between graduate preparation and clinical teaching in nursing. *Journal of Nursing Education, 36*(7), 317-322.

Johnson, S. (2002). Development of educator competencies and the professional review process. *Journal for Nurses in Staff Development, 18*(2), 92-102.

Johnston, S.R. (1996). Evaluating the effectiveness of faculty as group members. *Nurse Educator, 21*(3), 43-50.

Kanter, R. M. (1977). *Men and women of the corporation.* New York: Basic Books.

Kavoosi, M. C., Elman, N. S., & Mauch, J. E. (1995). Faculty mentoring and administrative support in schools of nursing. *Journal of Nursing Education, 34*(9), 419-426.

Kelly, C. (2002). Investing in the future of nursing education. *Nursing Education Perspectives, 23*(1), 24-29.

Kotecki, C., & Eddy, J. (1994). Developing an orientation program for a nurse educator. *Journal of Nursing Staff Development, 10*(6), 301-305.

Lane, A. (1996). Developing healthcare educators: The application of a conceptual model. *Journal for Nurses in Staff Development, 12*(5), 252-259.

Lindemann, C. (2000). The future of nursing education. *Journal of Nursing Education, 39*(1), 5-11.

Love, C. (1996). How nurse teachers keep up-to-date: Their methods and practices. *Nurse Education Today, 16*(4), 287-295.

Ludwick, R., Dieckman, B., Herdtner, S., Dugan, M., & Roche, M. (1998). Documenting the scholarship of clinical teaching through peer review. *Nurse Educator, 23*(6), 17-20.

Magnussen, L. (1997). Ensuring success: The faculty development plan. *Nurse Educator, 22*(6), 30-33.

McElroy, A. (1997). Developing the teachers' role: The use of multiple focus groups to ensure grassroots involvement. *Nurse Education Today, 17*(2), 145-149.

Morin, K.H. & Ashton, K.C. (1998). A replication study of experienced graduate nurse faculty orientation offerings and needs. *Journal of Nursing Education, 37*(7), 295-301.

Mundt, M. (2001). An external mentor program: Stimulus for faculty research development. *Journal of Professional Nursing, 17*(1), 40-45.

National League for Nursing. (2001). *Position statement on lifelong learning for nursing faculty.* New York: Author.

Nugent, K. E., Bradshaw, M. J., & Kito, N. (1999). Teacher self-efficacy in new nurse educators. *Journal of Professional Nurisng, 15*(4), 229-237.

Oermann, M. (1998). Work-related stress of clinical nursing faculty. *Journal of Nursing Education, 37*(7), 302-304.

Oermann, M. (1999). Developing a teaching portfolio. *Journal of Professional Nursing, 15*(4), 224-228.

Reeve, M.M. (1994). Development of an instrument to measure effectiveness of clinical instructors. *Journal of Nursing Education, 33*(1), 15-20.

Riner, M., & Billings, D. (1999). Faculty development for teaching in a changing health care environment: A statewide needs assessment. *Journal of Nursing Education, 38*(9), 427-429.

Sarmiento, T., Laschinger, H. K., & Iwasiw, C. (2004). Nurse educator's workplace empowerment, burnout, and job satisfaction: Testing Kanter's theory. *Journal of Advanced Nursing, 46*(2), 134-143.

Siler, B., & Kleiner, C. (2001). Novice faculty: Encountering expectations in academia. *Journal of Nursing Education, 40*(9), 397-403.

Smolen, D. (1996). Constraints that nursing program administrators encounter in promoting faculty change and development. *Journal of Professional Nursing, 12*(2), 91-98.

Vezina, M., Chiang, J., Laufer, K., Garabedian, C., Padre, H., & Sanders, N. (1996). Competency-based orientation for clinical nurse educators. *Journal for Nurses in Staff Development, 12*(6), 311-313.

Ward-Griffin, C. & Brown, B. (1992). Evaluation of teaching: A review of the literature. *Journal of Advanced Nursing, 17*(12), 1408-1414.

CHAPTER EIGHT

ENGAGE IN SCHOLARSHIP

Scholarship is an essential component of the nurse educator role and nurse educators must engage in those professional activities that systematically advance the science of nursing (Nelson, 2001; Silva, 1999) and the science of nursing education. According to Boyer (1990), faculty scholarship includes the scholarship of discovery, teaching, application, and integration. These four forms of scholarship are not mutually exclusive, but instead constitute an integrated approach to faculty work that supports learning (Dirks, 1998). Scholarship includes the dissemination of nursing knowledge through various means, such as presentations, publications, faculty practice, community service, academic teaching, and research. To engage effectively in scholarship, the nurse educator:

- Draws on extant literature to design evidence-based teaching and evaluation practices

- Exhibits a spirit of inquiry about teaching and learning, student development, evaluation methods, and other aspects of the role

- Designs and implements scholarly activities in an established area of expertise

- Disseminates nursing and teaching knowledge to a variety of audiences through various means

- Demonstrates skill in proposal writing for initiatives that include, but are not limited to, research, resource acquisition, program development, and policy development

- Demonstrates qualities of a scholar: integrity, courage, perseverance, vitality, and creativity

Review of the Literature

The majority of articles addressing the nurse educator competency of engaging in scholarship were discussion articles examining the dimensions of scholarship, particularly within the academic environment. Elberson and Williams (1996) conceptualized scholarship as being multidimensional, a perspective congruent with Boyer's Model of Scholarship (1990). Boyer's model is frequently cited in the literature as a framework for restructuring and supporting the various aspects of faculty scholarship in schools of nursing (Brown et al., 1995; Sneed et al., 1995; Starck, 1996; Wood et al., 1998).

The concepts of scholar, scholarly role, and scholarship appeared in many articles. A scholar is an individual who is "a thinker, one who conceptualizes the questions as well as pursues the answers" (Meleis, 1992, p. 328). Scholarly roles that have been identified for nurse faculty include researcher (Byrne & Keefe, 2002; Clifford, 1997), clinician (Tolve, 1999), and teacher (Bartels, 1997). Scholarship in nursing itself has been defined as those professional activities that systematically advance the art and science of nursing (Nelson; 2001, Silva, 1999) through the generation and communication of knowledge. It also has been defined as the acquisition of knowledge through study, gathering information, synthesizing ideas, and generating new meaning (Worrall-Carter, 1995).

A review of the literature on engaging in scholarship in the nurse educator role generated the following themes: components of scholarship; knowledge of educational theory, nursing practice, and research; characteristics of a scholar; and a continuum for professional growth as a scholar.

Components of Scholarship

The most frequently referenced and applied model of scholarship to professional development, particularly in the academic setting, is that of Boyer (1990). He conceptualized four types of scholarship: scholarship of discovery (research, systematic study, and investigation), scholarship of integration (interpreting, drawing together, and gaining new insight), scholarship of application (applying knowledge to important problems), and scholarship of teaching (investigating teaching and learning). Historically, the scholarship of discovery has received the greatest attention and recognition in the broad academic arena.

Although Boyer's model of scholarship is the seminal model that has been adopted in many academic environments, some in nursing have criticized it as being too narrow for a practice discipline in which scholars may be practitioners, theorists, researchers, and/or educators (Riley, Beal, Levi, & McCausland, 2002; Storch & Gamroth, 2002). Riley et al. (2002) asserted that in a practice discipline such as nursing, there is a "dynamic interplay of the intellectual and experiential components of knowledge" (p. 384), and, modifying Boyer's model, proposed that a universal holistic model of scholarship with four interconnected domains – knowing, teaching, practice, and service – would have more relevance. The scholarship of knowing links the scholarship of discovery with application, which is critical for a practice-based discipline. The scholarship of teaching addresses how to prepare practitioners for lifelong learning. The focus of the scholarship of practice is on the influence of the practitioner on knowing, teaching, and service. Lastly, scholarship of service, although generally less recognized, is a part of nursing's code of conduct, to reach out to society and the community. Storch and Gamroth (2002) reported on how a collaborative of nursing programs in British Columbia used Boyer's model of scholarship to define and evaluate faculty scholarship. They described an "expanded" model based upon Boyer's original work that cross-tabulated the four forms of scholarship with each other to form a 16-cell model. They found this model to be helpful in guiding their discussions about scholarship within the collaborative's nursing programs.

In another model, Roberts (1995) conceptualized the domain of scholarship in nursing to consist of three areas: theoretical scholarship, clinical scholarship, and research scholarship. Theoretical scholarship focuses on the theoretical aspects of the discipline for the development of nursing knowledge; it may or may not involve empirical research or direct clinical practice. Clinical scholarship links theoretical and research scholarship through application into practice; it is an activity that includes "informed, intelligent, and clinically grounded analysis" (Diers, 1995, p. 28). Research scholarship is the equivalent of Boyer's scholarship of discovery. Three significant points set forth by Roberts are that not all research is scholarship, not everyone is a researcher scholar, and the boundaries between these three areas of scholarship are fluid.

Elberson and Williams (1996) linked Carper's patterns of knowing (1978) with clinical scholarship and suggested that the pattern of empirics are connected to the scholarship of teaching through the imparting of knowledge of nursing science to students. When educators teach by bringing their own experiences and understandings to the teacher/learner context, what is conveyed is Carper's pattern of esthetics. In addition, Elberson and Williams also asserted that creative teaching strategies that are based upon adult learning theories are necessary to empower students and achieve clinical scholarship.

Several articles presented models of how various schools of nursing examined and framed scholarship and identified methods to assess and promote it (Nelson, 2001; Raff & Arnold, 2001; Storch & Gamroth, 2002). In one research-based article, Naddy (1994) discussed a descriptive research study exploring Boyer's four-dimensional model of scholarship in relation to nurse faculty role behaviors. Findings from the 398 faculty surveyed revealed that faculty role behaviors were characterized as a two-dimensional construct of discovery and dissemination of knowledge scholarship and teaching scholarship.

Knowledge of Educational Theory, Nursing Practice, and Research

As pointed out by Stevens (1999), the larger context of health care as well as the context of higher education have influenced and continue to influence nursing education. Thus, to be competent, the nurse educator must understand the scholarly aspects of the roles they assume, specifically, the teacher role, the researcher role, and the clinician role. Although the following discussion considers each role separately, there exists considerable overlap among these roles.

In the teacher role, the nurse educator must have knowledge of educational theory, curriculum design, and evaluation methods. Through research, practice, and dialogue, the educator can develop this knowledge base (Tanner, 2002). Boyer emphasized that "pedagogical procedures must be carefully planned, continuously examined, and relate directly to the subject matter taught" (1990, p. 24). To this end, Stevens and Cassidy (1999) advanced the concept of evidence-based teaching as a strategy of "continuous examination of pedagogy in nursing education" that "can be accomplished through research to discover effective, efficient means of teaching and correlates of learning" (p. 4), thus establishing the link between the teacher and researcher roles.

To create a science of nursing education and a scholarship of teaching, further research investigating innovative practices in schools of nursing must be encouraged and supported (Diekelmann, 2002; Diekelmann & Ironside, 2002). Drevdahl et al. (2002) put forth a model that used reflective inquiry and self-study as a framework for enhancing the teaching practices of educators and promoting the scholarship of teaching. This model places value on both pedagogical scholarship and teaching as a scholarly activity by integrating research and teaching.

Kreber (2001) proposed that the nurse educator should have knowledge that is focused on three elements: instruction, pedagogy, and curriculum. Instructional knowledge is knowledge that the educator must have about the various components of instructional design. Pedagogical knowledge is knowledge about how to facilitate student learning. Curricular knowledge is knowledge about the goals, purposes, and rationale that guide program and course design and sequencing.

In the researcher role, the nurse educator must have a grasp of various research methodologies. Discovery scholarship (Boyer, 1990) encompasses the use of systematic inquiry to create new knowledge as a basis for practice and teaching. The educator must engage in research that can guide or evaluate clinical practice, the educational process, or program outcomes. The synthesis of knowledge within and across disciplines to create new insights and patterns is also part of this role. The nurse educator uses knowledge gained from research, theory, and practice to optimize learning in the clinical and classroom settings. Through research, the educator can develop new models for nursing education (Elberson & Williams, 1996).

The clinician role of the nurse educator with respect to scholarship is less well articulated, even though some have argued that all nursing faculty have a clinical role due to the very nature of nursing (Wood et al., 1998). This role includes integrating evidence-based knowledge into practice, modeling excellence in clinical practice, and teaching others in the practice setting. Brown et al. (1995) equated this role to application scholarship wherein "competency within one's clinical arena is paramount" (p. 28). Therefore, educators must strive to maintain a comprehensive knowledge base and practice competence in their clinical specialty areas, including the identification of gaps in the body of knowledge related to nursing practice.

In a national survey of nursing faculty (N = 402) and deans (N = 170) that explored nursing scholarship and faculty practice, deans and faculty did not differ significantly in their responses to items about scholarship (Tolve, 1999). The major theme uncovered through an open-ended question on the survey was the role strain faculty experienced as they tried to balance all the components of scholarship – teaching, service, practice, research, and dissemination of their research. The findings from this study supported considering the faculty practice role to be a component of scholarship as long as scholarly outcomes are achieved.

Characteristics of a Scholar

The nurse educator must possess certain skills and attitudes, or predispositions, to be a scholar. The educator who is a scholar is able to think logically and critically, problem solve, communicate ideas effectively (Chinn, 1999), have an ongoing commitment to knowledge development and pursuit of learning, and hold particular values, such as humility, collaboration, commitment, spirit of inquiry, and persistence (Dreher, 1997). The qualities of a scholar include integrity, courage, perseverance (Glassick, Huber, & Maeroff, 1997), vitality, reflection (Bartels, 1997), and creativity (Nelson, 2001; Smith, 2002), which is a concept that surfaces in a number of references to scholarship (American Association of Colleges of Nursing, 1999; Duldt, 1995; Elberson & Williams, 1996; Lynton & Elman, 1987; Rawnsley, 2003; Silva, 1999). This is not surprising as a main part of discovery is the ability to be creative. In addition, nurse educators must demonstrate a commitment to service with a community orientation. Diekelmann (1997) and Diekelmann and Ironside (1998) extended the concept of community to nursing education as they proposed a new pedagogy for nursing education, community reflective scholarship, that promotes learning community partnerships among teachers, students, and clinicians.

Educators who are scholars also possess other characteristics. They are teachers and learners, and serve as role models and mentors (Brown et al., 1995; Duldt, 1995; McGivern, 2003; Meleis, 1992). They critique, utilize, and conduct research, and secure resources to support scholarly endeavors. Demonstrating skill in proposal writing is another characteristic of a successful scholar.

Some research studies have focused on what "being a scholar" means to faculty and the activities of successful scholars. In a phenomenological study using a hermeneutical approach, Diekelmann and Ironside (1998), asked five nursing faculty teaching in doctoral programs and 10 nurses who were enrolled in doctoral programs to share their experiences in becoming a scholar. The pattern of "preserving reading, writing, thinking, and dialogue," which is how faculty and students sustain these activities in meaningful or oppressive ways, emerged as significant practices of scholarship that must be nurtured and maintained. The authors contended that faculty and students should think about how "… reading, writing, thinking, and dialogue, as lived experiences, are inseparable and seamless as well as repetitious, ongoing, circular, and never ending" (p. 1353).

A survey of 41 nursing programs in the United States indicated that the dimensions of scholarship within these nursing programs included teaching research, conducting research, publishing, grant writing, presenting, and consulting (Dienemann & Shaffer, 1992). Successful scholars conduct research, publish, and present scholarly work (Hodges & Poteet, 1992). Recognizing constraints of workload and time on nursing faculty scholarly productivity, McVeigh et al. (2002) described a case study on the development of a publication syndicate of faculty in an Australian school of nursing to encourage writing for publication and to support faculty development. As members of the syndicate, faculty met together for 1 hour every 2 to 3 weeks to review and critique manuscripts. An increase in the number of publications and a sense of fellowship and community among faculty emerged as significant gains from this endeavor.

The characteristics of the international scholarly contributions of nursing faculty have also been examined, albeit in a limited fashion. In a survey to examine international scholarly activities between 1985 and 1995, Lusk and Lash (2002) asked United States nursing faculty to describe their scholarly activities abroad. They received 247 responses from faculty with international experience. The activities faculty were involved in were broad and diverse, and dependent upon the geographic region of the world in which the experiences occurred. These activities included research, clinical education, consultation, and service.

Continuum for Professional Growth as a Scholar

Boyer advocated that "the documentation of scholarship should be a 'moving picture', not a 'snapshot' [and] evidence should be gathered over time" (1996, p. 5). Thus, the form of scholarship in which nurse educators engage is likely to evolve throughout their careers as they move from novice to expert scholar. There is support in the literature for mentoring of the young scholar by an experienced scholar (Adderly-Kelly, 2003; Byrne & Keefe, 2002; Duldt, 1995; Kitzen, 1999; McGivern, 2003; Roberts & Turnbull, 2002).

Weston and McAlpine (2001) described a continuum of growth toward the scholarship of teaching that takes place in three phases. Phase I is focused on growth in one's own teaching and personal knowledge about teaching and learning. During this phase, the educator reads about teaching and learning, reflects on his or her own teaching, engages in institutional teaching development activities, tests out some innovations in teaching, and uses evaluation feedback to improve teaching. In Phase II, nurse educators dialogue with colleagues about teaching and learning while developing and exchanging ideas for improvement. This dialogue makes explicit their pedagogical content knowledge. Mentoring of other teachers in the discipline may occur during this phase and educators may also provide leadership in teaching within the discipline and the institution. There is growth of understanding of the complexity of teaching and learning. During Phase III, a comprehensive knowledge of the research and literature on teaching and learning is important. The educator develops scholarly knowledge about teaching and learning that has significance and affects the institution and the field. Publishing and making presentations about teaching, both theoretically and empirically based, are part of this phase. The educator may obtain funding for teaching and to support research on teaching using an approach to inquiry consistent with understanding teaching and learning (Weston & McAlpine, 2001).

It is clear from this description of growth as a scholar in teaching and learning that being an educator requires a commitment to lifelong learning and career development. Even experienced educators should have the opportunity and be expected to participate in professional development opportunities to continue to grow in their role as a scholar.

Identified Gaps in the Literature

There exists limited empirical research in the literature addressing nurse educator engagement in scholarship. Much of the literature addresses the application of Boyer's model of scholarship in nursing or the importance of scholarship. In recent literature, the scholarship of teaching has received greater attention than other areas of scholarship. Additional research that addresses the application and evaluation of new and innovative approaches to the domains of scholarship warrants exploration.

Priorities for Future Research

The following priorities for future research related to the educator competency, engaging in scholarship, are recommended:

- What are the expected outcomes of scholarship or scholarly activity for nurse educators as influenced by institutional setting and faculty rank?
- What is the relationship between faculty engagement in scholarly activities and student learning?
- What are the facilitators and barriers to faculty scholarship?
- What institutional resources are most effective for developing and supporting the scholarship of nurse educators?
- How is scholarly teaching similar to and different from competent or expert teaching?

References

Adderly-Kelly, B. (2003). Promoting the scholarship of research for faculty and students. *The ABNF Journal, 14*(2), 41-44.

American Association of Colleges of Nursing. (1999). Defining scholarship for the discipline of nursing. *Journal of Professional Nursing, 15*(6), 372-376.

Bartels, J. (1997). Understanding teaching scholarship – Beyond the dichotomization. *Journal of Professional Nursing, 13*(5), 278.

Boyer, E. (1990). *Scholarship reconsidered: Priorities of the professoriate.* Princeton, NJ: The Carnegie Foundation for the Advancement of Teaching.

Boyer, E. (1996). Clinical practice as scholarship. *Holistic Nursing Practice, 10*(3), 1-6.

Brown, S., Cohen, S., Kaeser, L., Levine, C., Littleton, L., Meininger, J., Otto, D., & Rickman, K. (1995). Nursing perspective of Boyer's scholarship paradigm. *Nurse Educator, 20*(5), 26-30.

Byrne, M., & Keefe, M. (2002). Building research competence in nursing through mentoring. *Journal of Nursing Scholarship, 34*(4), 391-396.

Carper, B. (1978). Fundamental patterns of knowing in nursing. *Advances in Nursing Science, 1*(1), 13-23.

Chinn, P. (1999). From the editor. Scholarship: The paradoxes of the 14 Cs. *Advances in Nursing Science, 22*(2), v-vi.

Clifford, C. (1997). Nurse teachers and research. *Nurse Education Today, 17*(2), 115-120.

Diekelmann, N. (2002). "She asked this simple question:" Reflecting and the scholarship of teaching. *Journal of Nursing Education, 41*(9), 381-382.

Diekelmann, N. (1997). Creating a new pedagogy for nursing. *Journal of Nursing Education, 36*(4), 147-148.

Diekelmann, N., & Ironside, P. (1998). Preserving writing in doctoral education: Exploring the concernful practices of schooling learning teaching. *Journal of Advanced Nursing, 28*(6), 1347-1355.

Diekelmann, N., & Ironside, P. (2002). Developing a science of nursing education: Innovation with research. *Journal of Nursing Education, 41*(9), 379-380.

Dienemann, J., & Shaffer, C. (1992). Faculty performance appraisal systems: Procedures and criteria. *Journal of Professional Nursing, 8*, 148-154.

Diers, D. (1995). Clinical scholarship. *Journal of Professional Nursing, 11*(1), 24-30.

Dirks, A. (1998). The new definition of scholarship: How will it change the professoriate? Retrieved from http://webhost.bridgew.edu/adirks/ald/papers/skolar.html

Dreher, M. (1997). President's message. Nursing science values. *Reflections, 23*(3), 4-5.

Drevdahl, D., Stackman, R., Purdy, J., & Louie, B. (2002). Merging reflective inquiry and self-study as a framework for enhancing the scholarship of teaching. *Journal of Nursing Education, 41*(9), 413-419.

Duldt, B. (1995). Scholarly inquiry and research. *Nurse Educator, 20*(1), 13-14.

Elberson, K., & Williams, S. (1996). Innovative strategies for promoting clinical scholarship: A holistic approach. *Holistic Nursing Practice, 10*(3), 33-40.

Glassick, C., Huber, M., & Maeroff, G. (1997). *Scholarship assessed: Evaluation of the professoriate.* San Francisco: Jossey-Bass.

Hodges, L., & Poteet, G. (1992). The first five years after the dissertation. *Journal of Professional Nursing, 8*(3), 143-147.

Kitzen, A. (1999). Guest editorial. The relevance of scholarship for nursing research and practice. *Journal of Advanced Nursing, 29*(4), 773-775.

Kreber, C. (2001). The scholarship of teaching and its implementation in faculty development and graduate education. In Kreber, C. (Ed.), *Scholarship revisited: Perspectives on the scholarship of teaching* (pp. 79-88). San Francisco: Jossey-Bass.

Lusk, B., & Lash, A. (2002). A decade of international activities by US nurse faculty: A descriptive analysis. *Nursing Outlook, 50*(4), 144-151.

Lynton, E., & Elman, S. (1987). *New priorities for the university : Meeting society's needs for applied knowledge and competent individuals.* San Francisco: Jossey-Bass.

McGivern, D. (2003). The scholars' nursery. *Nursing Outlook, 51*(2), 59-64.

McVeigh, C., Moyle, K., Forrester, K., Chaboyer, W., Patterson, E., & St. John, W. (2002). Publication syndicates: In support of nursing scholarship. *The Journal of Continuing Education in Nursing, 33*(2), 63-66.

Meleis, A. (1992). On the way to scholarship: From master's to doctorate. *Journal of Professional Nursing, 8*(6), 328-334.

Naddy, D.(1994). Applying Boyer's scholarship model to nurse faculty role behaviors. *Dissertation Abstracts International, 55*(06), 2158B. (UMI No. 9425324).

Nelson, M. (2001). A model for scholarship in nursing: The case of a private liberal arts college. *Nursing Outlook, 49*(5), 217-222.

Raff, B., & Arnold, J. (2001). Faculty development: An approach to scholarship. *Nurse Educator, 26*(4), 159-161.

Rawnsley, M. (2003). Dimensions of scholarship and the advancement of nursing science: Articulating a vision. *Nursing Science Quarterly, 16*(1), 6-15.

Riley, J., Beal, J., Levi, P., & McCausland, M. (2002). Revisioning nursing scholarship. *Journal of Nursing Scholarship, 34*(4), 383-389.

Roberts, K. (1995). Theoretical, clinical and research scholarship: Connections and distinctions. In G. Gray, R. Pratt, & J. Lawler (Eds.), *Scholarship in the discipline of nursing* (pp. 211-222). Melbourne: Churchill Livingston.

Roberts, K., & Turnbull, B. (2002). Scholarly productivity: Are nurse academics catching up? *Australian Journal of Advanced Nursing, 20*(2), 8-14.

Silva, M. C. (1999). The scholarship of teaching as science and as art. *Inventio: Creative thinking about learning and thinking.* Retrieved from http://www.doit.gmu.edu/Archives/feb98/msilva.html

Smith, L. (2002). Is this scholarship? *The Australian Electronic Journal of Nursing Education, 18*(1). Retrieved from http://www.scu.edu.au/schools/nhcp/aejne/vol8-1/refereed/smith.html

Sneed, N., Edlund, B., Allred, C., Hickey, M., Heriot, C., Haight, B., & Hoffman, S. (1995). Appointment, promotion, and tenure criteria to meet changing perspectives in healthcare. *Nurse Educator, 20*(3), 23-28.

Starck, P. (1996). Boyer's multidimensional nature of scholarship: A new framework for schools of nursing. *Journal of Professional Nursing, 12*(5), 268-276.

Stevens, K. (1999). Advancing evidence-based teaching. In K. Stevens & V. Cassidy (Eds.), *Evidence-based teaching. Current research in nursing education* (pp. 1-22). Sudbury, MA: Jones and Bartlett Publishers.

Stevens, K., & Cassidy, V. (1999). *Evidence-based teaching. Current research in nursing education.* Sudbury, MA: Jones and Bartlett Publishers.

Storch, J., & Gamroth, L. (2002). Scholarship revisited: A collaborative nursing education program's journey. *Journal of Nursing Education, 41*(12), 524-530.

Tanner, C. (2002). Learning to teach: An introduction to "Teacher talk: New pedagogies for nursing." *Journal of Nursing Education, 41*(13), 95-96.

Tolve, C. (1999). Nursing scholarship: Role of faculty practice. *Clinical Excellence for Nurse Practitioners, 3*(1), 28-33.

Weston, C., & McAlpine, L. (2001). Making explicit the development toward the scholarship of teaching. In C. Kreber (Ed.), *Scholarship revisited: Perspectives on the scholarship of teaching.* (pp. 89- 97). San Francisco: Jossey-Bass.

Wood, S., Biordi, D., Miller, B., Poncar, P., Snelson, C., Banks, M., Hemminger, S. (1998). Boyer's model of scholarship applied to a career ladder for nontenured nursing faculty. *Nurse Educator, 23*(3), 33-40.

Worrall-Carter, L. (1995). The emergence of a scholarly tradition in nursing. In G. Gray, R. Pratt, & J. Lawler (Eds.), *Scholarship in the discipline of nursing* (pp. 57-75). Melbourne: Churchill Livingston.

Creating an Evidence-based Practice for Nurse Educators

CHAPTER NINE
FUNCTION WITHIN THE EDUCATIONAL ENVIRONMENT

To be effective in their role, nurse educators must understand the educational environment in which they practice. They need to be knowledgeable about the history, culture, governing structure, and political dynamics that exist within the institution, as well as current trends in higher education and nursing education, since all these factors influence the faculty role. The educational environment is, in turn, influenced by political, economic, and social changes at the state, national, and international levels, and educators need to be aware of these external forces as well.

Nurse educators must also understand the mission of the institution and consider the compatibility of institutional mission and goals with their own personal philosophy, values, and goals. When determining if a particular institution is a "fit" with personal career goals, the nurse educator should consider the capacity of the position to meet her or his professional developmental needs and provide the necessary resources for supporting teaching, service, and scholarly activity.

It is also important for nurse educators to be able to function effectively in the political environment that exists within the educational setting in order to advocate for the nursing program and its needs within the institution, the higher education system, and other external constituencies. Political savvy is needed to meet the challenges of the faculty role, influence curricula, participate in institutional governance, and develop relationships within the institution and the community.

The following statements address the knowledge, skills, and attitudes nurse educators should acquire and use to work effectively within the educational environment. To effectively function within the educational environment, the nurse educator:

- Uses knowledge of history and current trends and issues in higher education as a basis for making recommendations and decisions on educational issues

- Identifies how social, economic, political, and institutional forces influence higher education in general and nursing education in particular

- Develops networks, collaborations, and partnerships to enhance nursing's influence within the academic community

- Determines own professional goals within the context of academic nursing and the mission of the parent institution and nursing program

- Integrates the values of respect, collegiality, professionalism, and caring to build an organizational climate that fosters the development of students and teachers

- Incorporates the goals of the nursing program and the mission of the parent institution when proposing change or managing issues

- Assumes a leadership role in various levels of institutional governance

- Advocates for nursing and nursing education in the political arena

Review of the Literature

Research literature about the educational environments in which nurse educators function is limited. Research studies that were found in the literature uncovered three primary themes: the organizational culture or work environment; professional goals and institutional "fit," and role negotiation within the educational environment. With respect to role negotiation, several works describing changes in the British system of nursing education are included in this review as they illustrate the impact of the higher education environment on the educator role.

Organizational Climate and Work Environment

The impact of the organizational climate and work environment on the educator role and productivity was examined by several authors. Hawks (1999) investigated faculty perceptions of organizational culture in schools of nursing, the empowering teaching behaviors used by faculty in these schools of nursing, and the relationships between the two. The study's conceptual framework was derived from Schein's concepts of organizational culture (as cited by Hawks) and the empowerment process. Instruments for this study included the Survey of Organizational Culture (SOC), which was used to measure faculty perception of organizational culture, and Part II of the Status and Promotion of Professional Nursing Practice Questionnaire (SPPNPQ), which was used to measure empowering teaching behaviors used by faculty. Reliability was established for both instruments and determined to be satisfactory. Findings were based on data from 281 nursing faculty employed in public, Research I institutions located within the North Central Association area. Although the majority of the nine subscale scores in the SOC instrument reflected neutral perceptions, three subscale scores reflected moderately positive perceptions. These positive perceptions were for orientation to customers, impact of mission, and managerial depth/maturity. Subjects reported using less than half the identified empowering teaching behaviors often in their own teaching. The authors cited this as a critical concern, but indicated that it was not known if this finding reflected a measurement issue or if faculty did not perceive themselves to be empowered. A major implication of this study is that educators may need to seek out a more empowering role within the organization for themselves so that they can create a more beneficial learning environment for students.

Two other studies addressed the climate in which nurse educators work. Lubbert (1995) investigated the organizational structure and climate in schools of nursing. A group of 111 full-time faculty from associate degree and baccalaureate programs was involved in the study. Climate was measured by a modified version of the Moos Work Environment Scale. The investigator explored relationships between centralization and perceptions of climate, formalization and climate, and vertical complexity and climate. A significant positive relationship was found between decentralization and a favorable climate. Faculty seemed to perceive a more favorable climate when responsibilities were clear and less supervision was present. In the second study, Doughty, May, Butell, and Tong (2002) asked a group of nursing faculty (N = 31) working in the same institution about their work environment. Expected and real faculty perceptions of their work environment were measured with two forms of the Moos Work Environment Scale. Reliability data for the scale were not provided for this study. A wider range of differences in "real" (actual) and expected scores was found in the measures of work pressure, physical comfort, and managerial control. Faculty reported more work pressure than they expected, a less pleasant physical environment than they expected, and less managerial control than they expected. It was not reported if these differences were statistically significant.

Mosser and Walls (2002) reported on a study that examined faculty perceptions of the relationship between the chairperson's leadership behaviors and organizational climate. The authors asserted that organizational climate is largely determined by the behaviors of leaders within the organization. Faculty respondents (N = 252) completed Bolman and Deal's Leadership Orientations Questionnaire and Borrevik's Organizational Climate Description Questionnaire-Higher Education. Satisfactory reliability and validity data were reported for both instruments. According to Bolman and Deal's leadership theory, leadership behaviors can be framed as structural, human resource, political, and symbolic. Borrevik asserted that organizational climate domains can be categorized as consideration (support for faculty), intimacy (social aspects of the organizational environment), disengagement (fractionalized faculty), and production emphasis (close supervision of faculty). Consideration and intimacy are considered to be characteristics of an open climate. Disengagement and production emphasis are marks of a closed organizational climate. About 60% of the faculty indicated that their chairs used one or more of the leadership frames as defined by Bolman and Deal. Respondents ranked the use of the leadership frames in order from most common to least common to be human resource, structural, symbolic, and political. Significant relationships ($p < .01$) were found between the human resource frame and consideration, the structural frame and production emphasis, the political frame and consideration, and the symbolic frame and consideration. There was a negative correlation between the four frames and disengagement. The findings of this study suggest that the leadership frames of administrators do influence the organizational climate and they should make a conscious effort to examine their leadership style. The authors identified study limitations to include the regional restrictions of the population, sample size, and the sole use of faculty perceptions without comparative data being obtained from administrators.

In a longitudinal study conducted over a two-year period, Fong (1993) investigated the relationships among overload, social support, and burnout. A sample of 140 faculty completed the first phase of the research, while 84 participated in both the first and second phases of the research. In addition to completing the Work Environment Scale, the Role Overload Scale (as cited in Fong, 1993), and the Maslach Burnout Inventory (as cited in Fong, 1993), subjects were asked about the number of hours worked, tenure status, and educational preparation. Job demands, time pressure, and the extent to which job inadequacy or role incompetence contributed to increased feelings of burnout or emotional exhaustion. Emotional exhaustion was accompanied by depersonalization of students and diminished feelings of accomplishment. Faculty perceived that department chair and peer support were positive factors in decreasing burnout, and achieving tenure appeared to improve the feeling of accomplishment. However, job demands continued to be a major source of burnout over the time of the study.

Research on organizational climate and work environment varies in methodology and factors studied. Overall, faculty seem to appreciate an environment that provides defined goals, but they also desire a degree of autonomy. Job demands are perceived as the major factor contributing to a more negative work climate.

Professional Goals and Institutional "Fit"

Studies about faculty recruitment and retention provide insights into the educational environment and the importance of achieving an institutional "fit" with one's professional goals. Froman (1996) investigated the importance of selected fixed and modifiable institutional characteristics in attracting experienced nurse faculty who had a record of research. The most important modifiable items that attracted senior faculty were research support, salary, and the potential for professional collaboration. Fixed characteristics, such as geographical location, were less important. These findings have implications for faculty recruitment efforts, and demonstrate the importance of being flexible with expectations, especially when trying to recruit expert faculty.

In a descriptive study focused on nurse practitioner (NP) faculty, Jones and Norton (1999) addressed faculty development and support needs. Nurse practitioner faculty (N = 128) completed a researcher-developed survey in which they identified the following issues that need to be addressed by administrators in order to retain qualified NP faculty: preparation of NP faculty for teaching, lack of administrator and colleague knowledge about NP practice requirements, salary, and difficulties implementing the research role. According to the authors, these specific needs and concerns of NP faculty must be addressed by the institution to maintain high quality practitioner education.

Job satisfaction is one measure of fit with the institution. Moody (1996) conducted a study of faculty in universities offering a doctoral degree in nursing. Thirty-five schools participated, from a total population of 44. Organizational characteristics and role orientation were studied in relation to job satisfaction variables. Job satisfaction was operationally defined as the "work itself, pay, opportunities for promotion, supervision, coworkers, and the job in general" (p. 272). Pay, level of students taught, and length of contract were positively related to job satisfaction. Time for scholarly activity and committee work outside the institution also were cited as contributing to job satisfaction.

Snarr and Krochalk (1996) also studied job satisfaction among nursing faculty. The purpose of their study was to examine the relationship between organizational characteristics such as work required by the job, pay, opportunities for promotion, extent of supervision, collegiality of coworkers, and faculty job satisfaction. Findings from 327 respondents indicated that nurse faculty were generally satisfied with their jobs and that there were no organizational characteristics that yielded a significant relationship with job satisfaction. One limitation of the study was that the researchers questioned the usefulness of the instrument (Revised Job Descriptive Index) used to measure job satisfaction among professional discipline faculty in academic settings. While the instrument itself has been found to be reliable with high levels of discriminant validity, it was standardized with industrial and corporate employees. The researchers recommended that the study be replicated to include dimensions of job satisfaction that are specific to the academic environment.

A meta-analysis of nurse faculty job satisfaction by Gormley (2003) considered six studies published between 1976 and 1996. Study variables were "professional autonomy, leader expectations, role conflict, role ambiguity, consideration of the leader, initiating structure behavior of the leader, organizational climate, and organizational characteristics" (pp. 175-176). Factors found to positively influence job satisfaction were leader expectations, consideration of the leader, and initiating structure behaviors in which the leader organizes activities. Role conflict and role ambiguity were included in only one study in this meta-analysis and were both reported to be negatively related to job satisfaction.

What do "peak performers" do differently in the education environment? Fong (1992) studied eight nurse educators identified as being "excellent." Using a qualitative approach, Fong interviewed the participants three times over an eight-year period. These educators identified the ability to set priorities, concentrate on self-mastery of their personal goals, and experience the rewards of teaching as being crucial in helping them be peak performers. Student expectations and university expectations of good teaching were important motivating factors as well.

Not surprisingly, novice educators' perceptions of the educational environment are different from the perceptions of the experienced educator. A qualitative study designed to ascertain the meaning of the new faculty experience indicated that the expectations of novice educators were not always addressed adequately (Siler & Kleiner, 2001). Four themes – expectations, learning the game, being mentored, and fitting – were found to describe the novice educator's experience. Study participants reported feelings, thoughts, and incidents related to unfamiliarity, incongruities, assistance from colleagues, trouble finding answers, performance concerns, and reflecting on their choice. The authors discussed several implications for creating an environment more conducive to the new faculty experience; for example, assigning teaching responsibilities that are a fit for the faculty's expertise and encouraging a mentoring relationship. It is important that the mentorship of new faculty continue for a sufficient time period to facilitate acclimation to the academic setting.

Morin and Romeo (1994) investigated the orientation needs of experienced undergraduate nursing faculty when they began new jobs. Factors studied were knowledge of the educational environment, academic environment, social milieu, political milieu, and campus geography. The factors deemed most helpful when transitioning to a new job were knowledge of the educational and academic environment, and orientation to the social milieu of the institution. Information about the educational environment included the curriculum and clinical learning as well as student evaluation and advisement. Role expectations and organizational structure were addressed in academic environment and social milieu.

A replication study by Morin and Ashton (1998) focused on experienced nurse faculty working in graduate programs. The same areas that were considered most helpful in the first study were also considered most helpful in the replication study. Respondents expressed the need for additional information about the social milieu, particularly about faculty networks and resources for scholarly activities. The researchers identified role strain as a barrier to pursuing scholarly endeavors in both studies.

As one would expect, the literature supports that nurse educators seek jobs that provide professional satisfaction. Institutional fit or satisfaction is largely dependent upon adequate pay, ability to meet one's own professional goals within the institution, collegiality and collaboration among coworkers, and adequate resources for achieving role expectations. The literature also documents the need for special attention to be given to novice faculty as they assimilate their role in academia.

Role Negotiation Within the Educational Environment

The role of the nurse educator has been greatly impacted by the many changes that are occurring in global health care delivery systems. The manner in which changes in health care have led to reform in nursing education are illustrated by studies from the United Kingdom and Australia (Cahill, 1997; Camiah, 1996; and Sellers & Deans, 1999). In response to health care demands in these countries, the educational environments in which nurse educators teach are being restructured and the roles and responsibilities of nurse educators are being renegotiated. Examples of nursing education reform have included moving nursing education into higher education systems, increasing emphasis on higher-order thinking skills, and incorporating managerial values and cultural concepts into the curriculum. For example, Camiah (1996) involved British educational nursing staff (N = 73) and service nursing staff (N = 42) in a mixed-method study designed to determine the major role and work changes that would be experienced by nurse tutors (educators) under the implementation of Project 2000. Project 2000 is a national nursing curriculum project implemented to better prepare graduates for practice in an increasingly complex U.K. health care system. Pertinent to this discussion of the educational environment were the changes perceived to be present in a new higher education setting. Changes identified in the role of the nurse tutors included the need for effective time management; new academic skills, including different teaching/learning strategies; and closer linkages to the service sector. A later study by Camiah (1998) focused on nurse lecturers and the changes in their clinical role. Observations and interviews over 2-5 years involved nursing lecturers and other health professionals (N = 41). The author noted the need for nurse lecturers to be more involved with the clinical aspects of teaching and to provide support for clinical nursing staff to facilitate a positive learning environment for students. A joint nurse teacher-practitioner role was recommended to improve nursing education.

Another British study by Cahill (1997) looked specifically at the role of nurse teachers functioning in a new higher education setting. Nurse teachers are expected to maintain teaching competence while balancing the demands for research and clinical practice activities. The author recommended that future studies focus on the workload requirements of the nurse teacher role to meet the multiple demands of the role and provide quality education.

In Australia, the movement of nursing education into higher education a decade ago is said to have advanced the nursing discipline. However, nurse educators in Australia (Sellers & Deans, 1999) are concerned about the future of this advancement of nursing as workforce demands increase. Nurse educator respondents (N = 369) in this study addressed issues of equal status in academia, the need for more resources, the increase in nurse educators' workload, and the need for a concerted, cohesive effort to foster quality nursing education. The authors called for increased collegiality among nurses in order to advance nursing science and the discipline, increase the quality of nursing education, and achieve parity with other disciplines in the academic environment.

A study by Congdon and French (1995) examined collegiality and adaptation among nursing faculty in the United Kingdom as nursing education moved from the National Health Service to higher education. Interviews with five nurse lecturers addressed aspects of developing collegiality and integration within a new educational environment. Themes that emerged from the interviews included concerns about in-groupism, or group cohesion; "nursing" or helping the students in the higher education environment; feelings of being different from other academics; and changes in power relationships from what had previously been experienced in practice settings. The authors indicated that adaptation needed to occur at both the personal and program level. Other issues discussed were the need for more integration into the academic setting, the use of adult learning strategies to promote independence of the students within the university setting, and the need for nurse educators to understand how to balance teaching demands with research and publication. The authors recommended devoting resources to assist nurse lecturers in making the adjustment to the higher education environment.

Brendtro and Hegge (2000) addressed the impending shortage of nurse educators in the United States. Using data from a statewide survey of nurses with graduate degrees that yielded a 61 percent return rate, the researchers noted nursing faculty are, on average, older than the general nurse population. Lack of competitive salaries in academia, the need to maintain one's clinical competence, and the demands of higher education were cited as reasons for nurses with higher degrees choosing not to pursue careers in academia. Difficulty in obtaining the appropriate education was reported as a problem relative to academic qualifications for nurse educators. The authors suggested that an examination of faculty roles, changing reward systems, and other strategies should be explored in order to meet the demand for nursing faculty. Limitations of this study included the fact that the respondents only represented nurses in one midwestern state and that those who chose to respond may have different perceptions from those who did not participate.

The studies cited for this competency mirror the current and lingering concerns of nurse educators in academic settings. Role expectations of academia coupled with the demands of a professional practice discipline require competence in the discipline, competence as educators, and an understanding of the educational environment in which one is employed. As greater numbers of experienced nurse educators retire and more novice educators enter the workforce, it will be essential that the nursing profession actively address the professional development needs of these educators to ensure that they will be able to achieve a "fit" and function effectively within the educational environment in which they teach.

Identified Gaps in the Literature

Research about nurse educators functioning effectively within the educational environment is minimal. Those studies reported in the literature have focused on organizational culture and its impact on faculty, and the importance of institutional fit with the educator's professional goals. Other studies in recent years have focused on the changing role of the nurse educator in other countries such as the United Kingdom and Australia and the emerging complexities of the role as a result of those changes. However, many elements of this nurse educator competency have not been studied directly.

Although research has addressed the organizational culture or work environments of nurse educators, the variability of research methodology and factors studied make it difficult to develop a body of knowledge in this area. Replication studies with nurse educators in a variety of educational settings are needed. Both replication studies and multisite studies would lead to further understanding of how nurse educators learn to function effectively in educational environments.

The importance of institutional fit for the nurse educator has been studied to some extent. As noted, a few studies have addressed areas such as recruitment and retention, job satisfaction, and role expectations. Additional studies are needed, especially in relation to novice faculty. Studies about role adaptation of new nurse educators moving into educational environments from practice environments would assist in determining the best practices associated with negotiating and facilitating the implementation of new faculty roles.

Priorities for Future Research

As noted, minimal investigation has been reported relative to the effective functioning of nurse educators in the educational environment. Research is needed to determine how to create the most favorable organizational culture or work environment for nurse educators to help them flourish in their educational career.

Additional investigation is needed about how to achieve institutional fit with one's professional goals as a nurse educator. Areas studied include recruitment and retention of faculty, job satisfaction, and role expectations, but we do not know what factors make a job attractive or how to match program goals with faculty strengths.

Nurse educators participate in a variety of activities connected to the governance of their institutions. Nurse educators' contributions to higher education and their ability to function effectively within the educational system are largely undocumented. Faculty and administrators outside the nursing discipline often comment on the strong work ethic of nursing faculty and the many positive contributions they make to institutional governance. Moving beyond such anecdotal evidence, empirical knowledge is needed to facilitate an understanding of the nursing faculty role within the academy, assist nurse educators to develop professionally within the institution and acquire the skills to assume leadership in institutional governance, and create an institutional environment that is conducive to faculty development and learning.

Areas for future research include, but are not limited to, the following:

- What systems and infrastructures facilitate effective implementation of all aspects of the nurse educator role in academia?

- What models or measures are useful in assessing nurse educator productivity?

- What are the experiences of new faculty with limited knowledge of the academic environment as they transition from a clinical role to an academic one?

- What are the contributions (e.g., institutional governance, faculty governance, institutional assessment) of nurse educators to the institution?

- What are the challenges faced by nurse educators who participate in institutional governance?

- How do nurse educators define a satisfactory work environment? How are these definitions similar to or different from educators in other disciplines?

- What are the challenges and strategies for negotiating the role demands of a practice discipline in an educational setting?

- How effective are nursing faculty in practicing within the political climate that characterizes academic institutions?

References

Brendtro, M., & Hegge, M. (2000). Nursing faculty: One generation away from extinction? *Journal of Professional Nursing, 16*(2), 97-103.

Cahill, H.A. (1997). What should nurse teachers be doing? A preliminary study. *Journal of Advanced Nursing, 26*(1), 146-153.

Camiah, S. (1998). Current educational reforms in nursing in the United Kingdom and their impact on the role of nursing lecturers. *Nurse Education Today, 18*(5), *368-379.*

Camiah, S. (1996). The changing role and work of British nurse tutors; A study within two demonstration Project 2000 districts. *Journal of Advanced Nursing, 23*(2), 396-407.

Congdon, G., & French, P. (1995). Collegiality, adaptation and nursing faculty. *Journal of Advanced Nursing, 21*, 748-758.

Doughty, J., May, B., Butell, & Tong, V. (2002). Work environment: A profile of the social climate of nursing faculty in an academic setting. *Nursing Education Perspectives, 23*(4), 191-195.

Fong, C.M. (1992). A model for peak performance. *Nurse Educator, 17*(4), 15-18.

Fong, C.M. (1993). A longitudinal study of the relationships between overload, social support, and burnout among nursing educators. *Journal of Nursing Education, 32*(1), 25-30.

Froman, R.D. (1996). Attracting an expert, or what nurses leaders look for in academic jobs. *Nursing Outlook, 44*(5), 239-242.

Gormley, D.K. (2003). Factors affecting job satisfaction in nurse faculty: A meta-analysis. *Journal of Nursing Education, 42*(4), 174-178.

Hawks, J.H. (1999). Organizational culture and faculty use of empowering teaching behaviors in selected schools of nursing. *Nursing Outlook, 47*(2), 67-73.

Jones, T., & Norton, D. (1999). Faculty development and support needs of nurse practitioner faculty. *Nursing Outlook, 47*(5), 209-218.

Lubbert, V.M. (1995). Structure and faculty perceptions of climate in schools of nursing. *Western Journal of Nursing Research, 17*(3), 317-327

Maslach, C. (1981). *Maslach burnout inventory.* Palo Alto, CA: Consulting Psychologists Press.

Moody, N.B. (1996). Nurse faculty job satisfaction: A national survey. *Journal of Professional Nursing, 12*(5), 277-288.

Morin, K.H., & Ashton, K.C. (1998). A replication study of experienced graduate nurse faculty orientation offerings and needs. *Journal of Nursing Education, 37*(7), 295-301.

Morin, K.H., & Romeo, K.C. (1994). Experienced faculty orientation offerings: Do they meet faculty needs? *Journal of Nursing Education, 33*(3), 125-131.

Mosser, N.R., & Walls, R.T. (2002). Leadership frames of nursing chairpersons and the organizational climate in baccalaureate nursing programs. *Southern Online Journal of Nursing Research, 2*(3). Retrieved from http://www.snrs.org/members/journal.html

Sellers, E.T., & Deans, C. (1999). Nurse education in Australian universities in a period of change: Expectations of nurse academics for the year 2005. *Nurse Education Today, 19*(1), 53-61.

Siler, B.B., & Kleiner, C. (2001). Novice faculty: Encountering academia. *Journal of Nursing Education, 40*(9), 397-403.

Snarr, C.E., & Krochalk, P.C. (1996). Job satisfaction and organizational characteristics: Results of a nationwide survey of baccalaureate nursing faculty in the United States. *Journal of Advanced Nursing, 24*, 405-412

CREATING AN EVIDENCE-BASED PRACTICE FOR NURSE EDUCATORS

CHAPTER TEN

CREATING AN EVIDENCE-BASED PRACTICE FOR NURSE EDUCATORS

Theresa M. Valiga, EdD, RN, FAAN
Chief Program Officer, National League for Nursing

Historically, individuals who wish to teach at the primary or secondary levels of education have been required to complete a program that prepares them both in their content area (e.g., science, social studies) and in teaching. Students who are "education majors" typically complete courses about the history of education, policies and practices related to education, and how students learn. They also are required to complete a supervised practicum where they teach under the guidance and direction of the practicing teacher, as well as their college professor. But no such expectations exist for those who wish to teach at the postsecondary level.

To date, most individuals teaching in colleges and universities have been appointed to faculty positions because they have earned the terminal degree in their field and are thought to be experts – or evolving experts – in that field (e.g., Renaissance literature, computer science). Search committees concern themselves with candidates' credentials, publications, grants, mentors, networks, and potential to secure funding for continued work in their field. While candidates often are expected to make a presentation to the search committee or full faculty, that presentation often is about their research, and it rarely is evaluated in terms of the individual's ability to explain concepts clearly, excite the learner about the topic, relate complex ideas, or stimulate learning. In other words, candidates for faculty positions in colleges and universities rarely are evaluated on their ability to teach, what they know about current research related to learning or current issues in higher education, or other pedagogical matters. This book on nurse educator competencies is an important step in changing the existing culture of the teaching abilities of faculty, and it is most timely.

In a recent article in the *Chronicle of Higher Education* (Brainard, 2007), it is noted that the United States continues to lose ground as the world leader in science, as China, India and other developing nations surpass us on many measures. While there is agreement that we should strive to maintain prominence in science, engineering, and mathematics, there is little consensus about how to achieve that goal. This article suggests that one way for the United States to remain competitive is to focus on how faculty can be more effective *as teachers*, educators who promote students' critical thinking skills and performance, minimize the traditional emphasis on memorization, and fully engage students in learning. Such a challenge requires that the academic community be clear about the competencies of educators, provide professional development resources to develop or enhance such competencies, and institute appointment, promotion, and tenure processes that acknowledge and, indeed, reward educator competencies.

Nursing has not been blind to this challenge. In 1992, Davis, Dearman, Schwab, and Kitchens wrote about competencies of novice nurse educators. They acknowledged the need to prepare faculty for the educator role itself, and reported that most graduate preparation programs in nursing focused on "advanced knowledge and skill in clinical nursing," a situation that remains 15 years later. Their findings indicated that most novice educators did not feel proficient in most of the competencies of teaching and concluded that "many novice nurse faculty are not educationally prepared for the faculty role" (p. 162).

The topic of nurse educator competencies continued to be addressed in a study of Norwegian nurse educators' opinions of the importance and application of different nurse educator competence domains (i.e., nursing competence, teaching skills, evaluation skills, personality factors, and relationships with students) (Johnsen, Aasgaard, Wahl, & Salminen, 2002). These researchers reported that, while faculty recognized the importance of competence in each domain, analyses showed "few and weak correlations" (p. 297) between ratings of importance and whether the competencies were actually carried out in practice. Findings repeatedly suggested that students' needs were not a high priority for teachers, that faculty competence as clinicians was valued more than their competence as educators, and that "the educators did not practice what they [said] was of importance in their teaching practice" (p. 300).

It is clear what colleges and universities want in new faculty (Adams, 2002). As an outgrowth of the work of the Preparing Future Faculty (PFF) program (Gaff, Pruitt-Logan, & Weibl, et al., 2000), the higher education community has become increasingly aware of the need to incorporate preparation for teaching and academic citizenship – as well as for research – into doctoral programs. It is becoming ever clearer that "knowledge of one's field is necessary but not sufficient" (Adams, 2002, p. v) if we wish to achieve excellence in the faculty role and provide exceptional learning experiences for students.

While the number of teacher preparation programs in nursing has grown in the last few years – largely in response to the nursing faculty shortage – they are still quite limited in number. One hopes, however, that with the clarification of nurse educator competencies outlined in this book, these programs will prepare graduates for the full scope of the faculty role and not repeat old forms of education. Indeed, Adams (2002) notes that "while the world of academe has changed dramatically over the last two decades, most graduate programs that prepare new faculty for their first academic positions have not" (p. 1). According to this author, there is adequate documentation to conclude that "research has clearly documented the impact of the mismatch between graduate training and the multiple academic responsibilities facing new faculty" (p. 1).

Research also has shown what it is that faculty must do if they are to be effective in facilitating student learning, evaluating what students have learned and how they have changed as a result of their educational experience, designing and implementing innovative curricula, being citizens of the academy, and helping students develop and internalize an identity as a member of a particular discipline (i.e., what it means to be a nurse, think like a nurse, view situations like a nurse, and so on). The extent of that research is documented in this book and provides a strong evidence base for the practice of teaching, particularly teaching nursing.

Research supports the conclusion that a primary role of faculty is to facilitate student learning (Competency #1) and that all the task statements listed for that competency are, indeed, critical if we are to create environments "in classroom, laboratory, and clinical settings that facilitate student learning and the achievement of desired cognitive, affective, and psychomotor outcomes" (NLN, 2005, p. 15). Based on the evidence provided in this book, there is no question that faculty must be skilled at "helping students develop as nurses and integrate the values and behaviors expected of those who fulfill that role" (NLN, 2005, p. 17), and that the task statements about facilitating learner development and socialization (Competency #2) are relevant.

Perhaps one of the most challenging aspects of the faculty role is the use of assessment and evaluation strategies (Competency #3) to "assess and evaluate student learning in classroom, laboratory and clinical settings, as well as in all domains of learning" (NLN, 2005, p. 18). This is documented to be a critical aspect of the faculty role, and it is essential that educators are competent in it. Likewise, it is the responsibility of faculty to design curricula and evaluate program outcomes (Competency #4) that "reflect contemporary health care trends and prepare graduates to function effectively in [today's complex, unpredictable, constantly-changing] health care environment[s]" (NLN, 2005, p. 19). As the research reported in this book shows, the complex work of curriculum development, implementation, and evaluation integrates many abilities that educators need to develop and continually refine.

While many would agree that teaching, evaluation, and curriculum development are key elements of the role of a faculty member, there may be less agreement about the need for faculty to be change agents and leaders (Competency #5) or able to function effectively within the educational environment (Competency #8). Some may think that it is the educational administrator (i.e., dean, director) who should be viewed as the change agent or leader for a school or that it is only the senior, tenured faculty who need to know how to be effective "citizens of the academy." The research reported in this book challenges these assumptions and documents the need for all educators to be prepared and willing to take on the responsibility of "creat[ing] a preferred future for nursing education and nursing practice" (NLN, 2005, p. 20) and to be "knowledgeable about the educational environments within which they practice and recognize how political, institutional, social and economic forces impact their role" (NLN, 2005, p. 23).

If one is to continue to be effective as a teacher, the research cited in this book supports the conclusion that one must pursue continuous quality improvement in the nurse educator role (Competency #6), recognizing that one's role as an educator is "multidimensional and that an ongoing commitment to develop and maintain competence in the role is essential" (NLN, 2005, p. 21). One aspect of the role that demands lifelong development is the engagement in scholarship (Competency #7). In the academic community, there is no doubt that scholarship is an expected and vital aspect of the faculty role. But the definition of the nature of "scholarship" needs to be broadened to incorporate the scholarship of teaching (Boyer, 1990), and faculty need to be expected to and rewarded for rigorously examining their teaching and that of others, exhibiting a spirit of inquiry about teaching and learning, and demonstrating "qualities of a scholar: integrity, courage, perseverance, vitality, and creativity" (NLN, 2005, p. 23).

Despite all we know about how to facilitate learning and how to effectively implement the full scope of the faculty role, many questions remain. The research questions posed at the end of each chapter in this book stimulate established and evolving nurse educator/scholars to continue to question their practice, develop the evidence base for that practice, and contribute to the development of the science of nursing education.

Creating an evidence-based practice for nurse educators, building the science of nursing education, and achieving excellence in nursing education (NLN, 2006) will occur when more and more individuals are prepared through graduate programs for the full scope of the faculty role and demonstrate competence in all aspects of that role. These goals will be achieved when a significant cadre of those practicing in the faculty role – an advanced practice role in our discipline – commit themselves to continual study of teaching and learning in nursing. As scholars, faculty will be expected to help identify priorities for research in nursing education, engage in critique of extant educational research, identify gaps in knowledge, conduct scholarly concept analyses of significant education-related concepts, test or apply research findings, and conduct systematic inquiry/research about the educational enterprise.

Outlining nurse educator competencies is a foundational step in achieving excellence in nursing education. Such competencies serve as the basis for the nurse educator certification examination (NLN, 2007) and, as noted, for building a science of nursing education. They guide faculty in designing and implementing innovations in nursing education that can transform the way individuals are prepared for their roles and lives as nurses. All these activities are essential if we are to achieve excellence in nursing education; thus, the nurse educator competencies described in this book are key to our continued success in preparing graduates who provide exquisite care, who make significant contributions to interdisciplinary collaborations, and who influence the future of the profession. They are, therefore, no small matter, as they help those in and outside the academic community understand the complexity of the educator role.

References

Adams, K. A. (2002). *What colleges and universities want in new faculty*. Washington, DC: Association of American Colleges & Universities.

Boyer, E. L. (1990). *Scholarship reconsidered: Priorities of the professoriate*. Princeton, NJ: Carnegie Foundation for the Advancement of Teaching.

Brainard, J. (2007). The tough road to better science teaching. *Chronicle of Higher Education, 53*(48), A16-A18.

Davis, D. C., Dearman, C., Schwab, C., & Kitchens, E. (1992). Competencies of novice nurse educators. *Journal of Nursing Education, 31*(4), 159-164.

Gaff, J. G., Pruitt-Logan, A. S., Weibl, R. A., & participants in the Preparing Future Faculty Program. (2000). *Building the faculty we need: Colleges and universities working together*. Washington, DC: Association of American Colleges & Universities.

Johnsen, K. O., Aasgaard, H. S., Wahl, A. K., & Salminen, L. (2002). Nurse educator competence: A study of Norwegian nurse educators' opinions of the importance and application of different nurse educator competence domains. *Journal of Nursing Education, 41*(7), 295-301.

NLN (National League for Nursing). (2005). The *scope of practice for academic nurse educators*. New York: Author.

NLN (National League for Nursing). (2006). *Excellence in nursing education model*. New York: Author.

NLN (National League for Nursing). (2007). Certification for nurse educators. Retrieved from http://www.nln.org/facultycertification/index.htm.

CONTRIBUTORS

Wanda Bonnel, PhD, RN
Associate Professor
University of Kansas School of Nursing
Kansas City, KS

Barbara Chamberlain, DNSc, APN, C, CCRN, WCC
Corporate Director of Education and Research
Kennedy Health System
Cherry Hill, NJ

Pauline McKinney Green, PhD, RN
Professor
Howard University Division of Nursing College of Pharmacy,
Nursing and Allied Health Sciences
Washington, DC

Judith A. Halstead, DNS, RN, ANEF
Executive Associate Dean for Academic Affairs
Professor
Indiana University School of Nursing
Indianapolis, IN

Karolyn Hanna, PhD, RN
Professor
School of Nursing
Santa Barbara City College
Santa Barbara, CA

Carol Heinrich, PhD, APRN, CNE
Assistant Professor
School of Nursing
University of North Carolina - Wilmington
Wilmington, NC

Barbara J. Patterson, PhD, RN
Professor
School of Nursing
Widener University
Chester, PA

Elizabeth N. Stokes, EdD, RN, CNE
Professor
Department of Nursing
Arkansas State University
Jonesboro, AR

Jane Sumner, PhD, RN, APRN, BC
Associate Professor
School of Nursing
Louisiana State University Health Sciences Center
New Orleans, LA

Helen J. Streubert Speziale, EdD, RN, CNE, ANEF
Associate Vice President of Academic Affairs
Professor, Nursing Department
Misericordia University
Dallas, PA

Cesarina Thompson, PhD, RN
Chairperson & Professor
Department of Nursing
Southern Connecticut State University
New Haven, CT

Diane M. Tomasic, EdD, RN
Professor of Nursing
Nursing Program
West Liberty State College
West Liberty, WV

Patricia K. Young, PhD, RN
Professor
Minnesota State University, Mankato
School of Nursing
Mankato, MN

CREATING AN EVIDENCE-BASED PRACTICE FOR NURSE EDUCATORS